101

FREEDOM EXERCISES

A Christian Guide
for Sexual Addiction Recovery

Second Edition

Douglas Weiss, Ph.D.

Discovery Press

CONTENTS

PART TWO: PERSONAL GROWTH FREEDOM TECHNIQUES

PART THREE: MAINTAINING FREEDOM TECHNIQUES

APPENDIX

INTRODUCTION

101 Freedom Exercises: A Christian Guide for Sexual Addiction Recovery has been written for Christians who struggle with sex addiction and desire techniques to assist them throughout the different development stages of their recovery. As a recovering sex addict with over twelve years of successful recovery, my personal recovery journey has educated me immensely about the recovery process. I personally have practiced many of the exercises in the pages ahead. Additionally, as a therapist, researcher, author, and lecturer on the subject of sexual addiction, I have compiled these exercises and principles which have successfully helped many addicts to begin and maintain their freedom from sexual addiction.

These exercises are in the chronological order recommended for the progression of the sex addict's recovery. The journey of recovery teaches us "first things first." I encourage you not to pick and choose which exercises you will or will not do, but rather receive from each exercise the insight it has to offer as you complete the exercise.

This book can most certainly be used in conjunction with therapy or as part of 12 step or church support group. My hope is that you receive the precious gift of recovery that Jesus Christ has to offer as I have, and maintain it the rest of your life for your benefit and for the benefit of others.

If we can be of any service along the way, feel free to write to Heart to Heart Counseling Centers, P.O. Box 16716, Fort Worth, TX, 76162-0716 or call 817-377-HART (4278). You can also visit our website at www.sexaddict.com. Some of our materials include books, videos and cassettes related to sexual addiction as well as video therapy & education. Support products are also available for wives in a relationship with a sex addict. Telephone counseling is available for those not in the Fort Worth, Texas area. We are available as well to ministering to the church body, training seminars and men's meetings. For more in-depth services see the appendix of this book. We look forward to helping you become and stay free from sexual addiction. If God calls you into this ministry of healing and you would like to begin a freedom group in your church, see the appendix of this workbook on how you can start a freedom group. If you do start a group, please let our offices know so that we can refer those to you that call us and are in need of a group.

Douglas Weiss, Ph.D.

PART ONE:
BEGINNING FREEDOM TECHNIQUES

EXERCISE # 1

<u>DAILY TIME FOR RECOVERY</u>

Recovering from sexual addiction will be one of the hardest undertakings of an addict's life. The typical sex addict in the midst of his addiction, has clocked in hundreds and sometimes thousands of hours of repetitive sexually addictive conditioning. Many sex addicts rely heavily upon their sexual acting-out as a primary coping mechanism before beginning the journey of recovery.

Recovery is hard work and more importantly it is consistent work. Remember it took consistent behaviors to spiral you into your addiction. It only makes sense that consistent work is going to be a big part of recovery and reconditioning yourself into a life of freedom from sexual addiction.

In light of this, daily you are going to need time to practice many of the exercises in this workbook that will enhance your recovery process. These exercises have been successfully proven to work but only if you take the time to do them. This is consistent with the fact that in most areas of life, what you put into something, is also what you get out. So, you may need to get a daily calendar and try to come up with at least 15-30 minutes daily to work on your recovery from sexual addiction. This effort will make a big difference on how long it will take you to experience freedom. This of course is not the total amount of time you will need in working your recovery as we will discuss later about attending support groups. Scheduling these support group meetings on your calendar will also be a <u>very</u> important part of your freedom from sexual addiction!

My daily time for recovery is from ___6 PM___ to ___6:30___ .

_____
Your signature

_____
Wife's Signature (if applicable)

EXERCISE # 2

CLEANING HOUSE

The information in this exercise may be obvious to many Christian sex addicts but for the benefit of those who have never read anything about getting free from sexual addiction, this exercise must be discussed. "Cleaning house" at the beginning of your recovery will steer you from keeping that "one" magazine, video, or telephone number that could possibly cause you to relapse down the road. Many sex addicts that I have counseled with had their first relapse with "the one I didn't throw away."

To prevent this experience from happening later, it is imperative to throw away (don't try to sell or inflict this material on anyone else) any item that could cause you to relapse. For some sex addicts, this will be a magazine, a video, an article of clothes or possibly a computer disk.

To clean house a bit further, you may want to consider canceling cable television, internet access, magazine subscriptions or any other material that could be a threat to your sobriety during the first 90 days of freedom.

In the beginning of your recovery, it is much better to err on the side of being too cautious than to err on the side of not being cautious enough. Some of the more restrictive boundaries can be changed to less restrictive in the future when your recovery is not as fragile as it is in the beginning.

This exercise can be a great beginning for your recovery. If you feel you need help, you may want to ask a friend or support group member who has some stable sobriety if they can be supportive through this exercise. For some sex addicts, cleaning house is a new beginning. It's a time you mark as the beginning of your journey. This is a great way to start your recovery and remove some of the possibilities for future stumbles.

The date I totally cleaned house was _4-4-06_____.

EXERCISE # 3

<u>EARLY PRAYER</u>

Prayer is something that many sexual addicts find difficult to do, especially if they have avoided God because of the shame and guilt of their behavior or possibly what was done to them in the past. Prayer is simply a behavior that when put in place, can change the addict's disposition. We know from other addictions that an addiction is basically self-will run riot. This expression of addiction is basically "doing your own thing" which is not very helpful for the Christian sex addict's recovery.

Take time out to pray first thing in the morning. If you need help, just use the guidelines of the Lord's prayer. Don't forget to ask Jesus during your prayer time to help you stay sober, accountable and honest today so that you can stay free from sexual addiction. He is proud of you for starting your recovery. His death purchased your freedom. Your prayer can help you to realize this on a daily basis.

Prayer is a way for you to behaviorally change yourself. Sexual addiction for many addicts starts early in the day. Not necessarily the first thing in the morning, but maybe in the shower, on the way to work, or while driving. <u>Prayer is preventative</u>. It is a way of acknowledging that you are a sexual addict and are in desperate need of Christ's freedom. Without sobriety, the addict is on a path of self-destruction, not only in his own life but more than likely those around him have been devastated, either through his anger, depression or acting-out behavior.

The addict is in a fight every day, especially the first thirty to ninety days. The first thirty to ninety day period is the toughest part of recovery for the sexual addict so make sure you connect with Jesus. Your prayer doesn't have to be long. Prayer may or may not make you feel better instantly, but it is one of the Five Commandments (which we will be discussing in a later exercise) and if you begin to apply them to your life, you will begin to reap the benefits. As a Christian, prayer is one of the many tools that you can have in your search for freedom from sexual addiction.

The time in the morning I can pray is __6:45__ .

EXERCISE # 4

<u>READING RECOVERY MATERIAL</u>

Reading recovery material that is specifically related to sexual addiction is so important. There are currently several Christian books on the market addressing sexual addiction. It is very important to read some recovery material every day.

It is best to read in the morning. Addicts need to be reminded of what may be in store for them that day. Sometimes the recovery thoughts that you have just read about are the very tools that will get you out of a tough situation, such as a fantasy, and that will give you the strength to fight for your recovery that day. It is important that you involve your mind during your journey for freedom. It alone is not going to save you, but it may get you to behave so that you can maintain your abstinent behaviors and not pass your bottom line. A list of reading materials is provided in an exercise you will be reading about later.

By now you probably get a feeling that your morning is going to change. This can take five to fifteen minutes, and will make a dramatic change in your day. You are worth getting the freedom you need so that you can restore yourself, your family and friends. You are going to learn a lot, not only about yourself, but also about recovery in general so that you can get a picture of hope to integrate into a life-style of sobriety.

Reading your Bible is great to do on a daily basis. As a Christian, this will strengthen your spirit. Reading the Bible is not a substitute for educating yourself about sexual addiction. Ignorance regarding sexual addiction has probably cost you a lot of guilt and shame already. Informing yourself about it is a responsible behavior, such as a diabetic would study up on diabetes. Daily recovery reading is critical especially in the first ninety days of your recovery.

My daily reading time will be _6:30_.

EXERCISE # 5

<u>CALL SOMEONE</u>

A phone call can be the very thing that may save you from an acting-out experience today. The first step of the Twelve Steps talks about the word "we." "We" means that you need some one else in your program to help you. In the past, "I" has been the biggest focus in the addict's world. Previously the sex addict didn't have the resources to get help due to his powerlessness. In being powerless, sex addicts couldn't fight sexual addiction alone. What the addict can do is involve others in the fight to dissipate the energy that comes against his life to destroy it. Sexual addiction can not be dealt with alone. I have not experienced nor have I known any one else who has experienced freedom from sexual addiction <u>ALONE</u>.

As a Christian, you know the body has many parts. You need another person to be accountable to and check in with. Remember James 5:16, "...confess your faults...so you may be healed." The reverse is also true. Keep your faults (secret thoughts, behaviors) to yourself, and you **will** stay sick! Many sex addicts have years of research on staying sick. You must push past your comfort zone to get and stay healthy. There are no lone rangers in the Christian walk and there are definitely no lone rangers in achieving freedom from sexual addiction. Remember if you humble yourself, you can be free. If you do not, humiliation will await you whether anyone finds out about your behavior, or not.

A life-style of sobriety is a much greater goal than just being abstinent. There are several ways to address this *commandment* about making phone calls. One way is to wait until you get into crisis and then call someone to help you. This method does not work because if you don't have a relationship with anyone, you are putting up a barrier that could isolate you. Making a phone call and saying "I am a sex addict," is a big enough task all by itself to accomplish let alone having to tell someone you have never talked to before that you are close to acting out sexually.

When you are not alone, you are accountable. The way to begin making phone calls is to make one call in the morning to another recovering sex addict. Tell them that you are not in trouble but if you get in trouble, you are going to call someone today. If you are checked in with someone eventually the phone calls are going to turn into conversations that develop healthy relationships.

I used isolation during my past sexual addiction acting-out days and kept very few relationships that were not sexual. Sex addicts need relationships. Part of your re-socialization is making phone calls, feeling connected, and getting acceptance right at the beginning of the day. If you can make a phone call early in the morning to someone else in the program, you are going to find strength in your day. Like prayer, the phone is a tool you can use to help yourself get stronger especially within the first 30-90 days during when you are going to need other people to help you more than ever before. The people you call will benefit just as much if not more than you will, when you call them. Make a phone call every day. You don't need to philosophically agree with this concept or have a good feeling about it to decide if you are going to do it. This phone call behavior is so that you can get free today.

I will call _____(name) at _____(time).

EXERCISE # 6

<u>GOING TO SUPPORT GROUPS</u>

In Alcoholics Anonymous, there is an old expression that says, "There are three times when you should go to a meeting, 1. When you don't feel like going to a meeting, 2. When you do feel like going to a meeting and, 3. at Eight O'clock." It is not a matter of how you feel about it. It is how you behave about it. In Twelve Step meetings, there is a "ninety meetings in ninety days" principle. This principle is ideal. I know that in most major metropolitan areas, there are meetings every day of the week. This can be more difficult if you get into a tough situation when you are far removed from metropolitan areas. If this happens to you, you may want to consider talking with someone in a meeting about getting together with them more frequently as an option. There are Christians in many of these meetings. Heart to Heart Counseling Center has started *Freedom Groups* for churches with Christians struggling with sex addiction. If you are interested in starting a Freedom Group in your church, please contact us so that we can refer people to your group. See our Freedom Group information in the Appendix section of this workbook. If it isn't possible to start a Freedom Group and there none available in your area, you may have to attend a traditional support group also listed in the back of this workbook in the Appendix section. It is our belief that God wants to use His church to heal those struggling with sexual addiction in the church as well as in the community. If the church will open their healing doors, I believe we will see no less than a revival!

These meetings are basically to support you and at some point give back to others what you have learned through your own particular journey of recovery. Being around other recovering sex addicts is going to help you. First it is going to give you hope as you see other sex addicts having successful sobriety. Second, you may believe that if they can do it, you can too. You can learn things from them that they have learned through negative or positive experiences. I want to encourage you to go to as many meetings as possible.

The meetings I will make are:

Day _____   Time _____

Day _____   Time _____

Day _____   Time _____

Day _____   Time _____

Day _____   Time _____

Day _____   Time _____

Day _____   Time _____

EXERCISE # 7

EVENING PRAYER

Praying again in the evening may sound redundant. You can read *Exercise #3, Early Prayer* again to be reminded that this is not something you have to like or even agree with. Prayer is something that is best to do twice minimally every day. At the end of the day, if you are sober, thank God for keeping you sober that day. Every day of freedom is a miracle to personally thank Jesus for.

Freedom from sexual addiction isn't something you do by yourself. It is something you do with the help of God and others. If there are any other issues from the day you want to talk to God about, you can also bring them up at this time. Inquire if you don't have a relationship with God, and ask Him to open your relationship up and to send people to you to bring this about. It is important to begin and end your day in a spiritual place. The recovery program that is going to work is spiritual in nature. So, it is important to reestablish your own spirituality since you were born spirit, soul, and body. Many sex addicts don't nurture their spiritual component even though they are Christians. Make this a time of being thankful that you had a day of freedom. Even the worst day in recovery, is something to be thankful for. Even your best day without freedom you were covered with shame, guilt and fear. So, if you have any relief from those feelings, I believe it is appropriate to respond in prayer.

EXERCISE # 8

THE FIVE COMMANDMENTS
A Ninety-Day Check List

Freedom from sexual addiction has some basic principles that when applied, help the sexual addict sustain his recovery program. Early recovery is not simply understanding the facts nor is early recovery simply talking about sexual addiction. Recovery goes much deeper than simply talking about what was done in the past. Many Christians may talk about getting better. The Prodigal Son (who was probably a sex addict) did not get better or restored when he realized he was in bad condition. He had to consistently walk back to get the blessings of his freedom after weeks or months of walking. Then the party started — not before.

The Five Commandments are simple and can be put up on your wall or mirror at home. Write the commandments down and check off if you have done them today, this week, this month, and the first 90 days. The behavioral checklist can assure you that you are putting behavioral steps toward recovery as opposed to just coming to an understanding about sexual addiction. Coming to an understanding is not the only answer for the addict. You may have been in pain for years and years and possibly have had behaviors that have been repeated hundreds of times. It is for this reason that the Five Commandments, when put in place, can give you an action plan so that you can begin to arrest the addiction that you may have been struggling with for so long.

Simply put, the Five Commandments are the last five behaviors you have read in Exercises #3-#7. These Five Commandments are simple:

1. Pray in the morning.
2. Read recovery literature daily.
3. Call someone in recovery daily.
4. Meetings - Attend Twelve-Step Meetings or Freedom Groups.
5. Pray again, and thank God for sobriety.

The check list on the following page will help you monitor your behaviors toward recovery. Remember only believe your **behaviors** when it comes to recovery. Don't talk yourself into believing that if you **feel** free, you are. **Behave** free and you will be.

90 Day Check List

DATE	PRAY	READ	CALL	MEET	PRAY		DATE	PRAY	READ	CALL	MEET	PRAY
1							46					
2							47					
3							48					
4							49					
5							50					
6							51					
7							52					
8							53					
9							54					
10							55					
11							56					
12							57					
13							58					
14							59					
15							60					
16							61					
17							62					
18							63					
19							64					
20							65					
21							66					
22							67					
23							68					
24							69					
25							70					
26							71					
27							72					
28							73					
29							75					
31							76					
32							77					
33							78					
34							79					
35							80					
36							81					
37							82					
38							83					
39							84					
40							85					
41							86					
42							87					
43							88					
44							89					
45							90					

EXERCISE # 9

<u>MAXIMIZED THINKING</u>

The maximized thinking technique is easy to understand. Simply ask yourself daily, (especially during the first year of recovery); "Is this the most I can put into my recovery today?" If the answer is more "yes" than "no," you will find yourself progressing through recovery quite well. Maximized thinking plays a big part in early recovery.

Those who consistently maintain the Five Commandments (which you learned about in the previous exercise) as much as possible, will make tremendous gains with maximized thinking added to their personal, spiritual, sexual and financial lifestyle. I have seen many sex addicts who have chosen maximized thinking in their recovery who have doubled their income in their first year as well as experienced a much healthier social, spiritual and sexual life-style.

Other options are shades of *minimized* thinking which is asking yourself "how little can I do" to recover in order to show others you are trying. This type of minimized thinking is done mostly on a less than conscious level and can be measured by a lack of recovery behaviors.

One way I determine the sex addict's level of seriousness in early recovery, is by his recovery behaviors. Intention, no matter how good, misleads you to think that you are in recovery when you actually are not. The Five Commandments is a good way to determine if you are applying maximized thinking or some other approach to what may be the hardest task of your life, that being recovery from sexual addiction. If you are still reading up to this point, that is a good sign, but keep on going! Your life can be 10 to 100 times better than any day living actively in a sex addicted lifestyle. Trust me when I say "you are worth your recovery," but nobody deserves their freedom from sexual addiction without effort, and nobody that I know gets it that way either. So, maximize the early part of your recovery, and you will have the rest of your life to thank yourself for the time you put into the beginning of your freedom journey.

Remember that you have not resisted sin unto death as Christ has for us. Think, "What is the best I can do to get and stay free for Him, since he has given His best for me."

EXERCISE # 10

RETRAINING THE BRAIN

As a sex addict, your brain has been conditioned neurologically to your acting-out behaviors. Many sex addicts were exposed to pornography at a young age and began to masturbate and/or fantasize with it. Every time the addict ejaculated, he sent a rush of chemicals to his brain called endorphins and enkephalins. The brain, as an organ of the body, has no morality. It just knows that when it gets a rush of what I call brain "cookies," or chemicals, it feels good. The rush could be from heroin, sky diving, sex or cocaine, but whatever has caused the rush, the brain, as an organ would not have a moral dilemma on how it got this rush.

After frequent ejaculations brought on by acting-out, the sexual addict begins to develop neurological pathways in the brain while acting out sexually. The brain as an organ, adjusts to getting it's neurological need met by the cycle of going into a fantasy state and minutes later sending the brain a rush of "brain cookies" through ejaculation.

To recover from sexual addiction, you must retrain your brain to not connect the fantasy world with these so called "brain cookies." To stop this biological cycle that the sex addict had set up (anywhere from 10 to 50 years), he will need a biological reconditioning cycle. One way is to place a rubber band on either wrist and when you start to have sexually inappropriate thoughts, snap the rubber band on the inside of your wrist. This sets up a cycle in your brain that says "fantasy = pain" instead of "fantasy = pleasure." The body is designed to avoid pain, and so this will reduce the amount of fantasies that you are having and eventually lessen the inappropriate thoughts so that you can focus on your freedom. You can memorize and quote appropriate scriptures to strengthen your spirit when you snap the rubber band, but use the rubber band to recondition your brain.

The average person who is very consistent with this reconditioning exercise of the brain finds about 80% of the fantasy life-style subsides within the first thirty days and if continued throughout the first 90 days, they find intruding thoughts are minimal and manageable with other exercises discussed later. This is a great exercise to truly "take your thoughts captive." You deserve a clean thought life and a retrained brain, and with consistency, you can achieve it. This exercise is a very effective tool for the early part of your freedom from sexual addiction.

I placed the rubberband on my wrist _____.
(Date)

EXERCISE # 11

<u>BEGINNER'S BIBLIOTHERAPY</u>

The following books and workbooks will be helpful in your early recovery from sexual addiction. (See Appendix for descriptions.)

<u>RELIGIOUS TITLES</u>	<u>AUTHOR</u>	<u>PRICE</u>
The Final Freedom (book/audio series)	D. Weiss	$22.95/35.00
101 Freedom Exercises	D. Weiss	$39.95
Steps to Freedom	D. Weiss	$14.95
Faithful and True	M. Laaser	$14.95

<u>TRADITIONAL TITLES</u>	<u>AUTHOR</u>	<u>PRICE</u>
The Final Freedom	D. Weiss	$22.95
Out of the Shadows	P. Carnes	$14.95
Hope and Recovery	Comp Care	$14.95
Sex and Love	Griffin-Shelly	$29.00

EXERCISE # 12

THE THREE-SECOND RULE

The three-second rule is simple but when applied, can stop the Christian sex addict from beginning a fantasy before it happens. If you are looking at someone in an inappropriate manner, count to three and then turn away, and DON'T look back! This works great, especially in public places like malls, restaurants or driving.

The "no turning back" is the hardest part. But, if you stick with this, it is easier for fantasies to subside and it reduces the cruising around "for a better look" or making contact with the person. In a way, this is rubbernecking in reverse. Instead of stretching to see what or who you are looking at, you count to three and stretch your neck to look at something else in the other direction that is safer for you and your freedom from sex addiction. This will probably add lots more time to your schedule too!

I have heard some addicts say they can only count to one and they have to look away. Do whatever you have to do to personalize this exercise to work best for you in order to stay free.

EXERCISE # 13

PRAY FOR THOSE WE OBJECTIFY

When you look at someone other than your wife in a sexual way, you are objectifying that person. It may be helpful to begin to see this person as someone who has feelings and is a person God loves. Think about this individual in a different light where they may have children and/or parents who love them. They may have been badly hurt by someone in the past. They are not cars that you can look at and compare shapes and proportions in order to determine their value. Nor are they some picture to be scanned into your "video" world in your mind so that you can manipulate them into your sexual fantasy world.

If you can pray for them and ask God to protect them or their spouse or children, it will allow you to put them in a relational context instead of an object context. This prayer may help you break up the fantasy otherwise known as the "bubble" of addiction before it fully forms around you. It may actually give your mind the freedom to get back to healthier thinking. Remember that the individuals that you objectify are persons God created, and He thinks highly of them.

Those of you who are fathers of little girls know how would you feel if you saw someone looking at your precious child in an impure manner. You would probably first feel sick and then angry. Remember, God is the father of the individual you are looking at, and no matter how old or attractive they are, God has feelings also about that person. So, pray for them and you will be on the right side of God.

EXERCISE # 14

<u>LOOKING THEM IN THE EYES</u>

Many male sex addicts have trouble looking a woman in the eyes because of years of conditioning and ejaculating to the female figure often portrayed in pornography. Videos, movies, and magazines sell this "object" and actually condition men to look at a female body first. Looking at a woman in an objectifying manner is a conditioned response. If you look her in the eyes it can keep you from scanning her as you would an object that you might purchase.

To keep eye contact while talking to a woman may be difficult at first because of your own guilt, shame or lack of self-esteem, but doing this can make it harder for you to start fantasizing since you are being looked back at directly. Additionally, looking your wife in the eyes during a sexual experience will also help you stay more relational and you will experience her as a person, not an object. Hopefully this is a person you would not want to hurt by fantasizing about. Remember eyes first and stay there, it can keep you from further trouble.

EXERCISE # 15

<u>TRIGGER GROUPS</u>

As you develop in your recovery, you may find that you have in the past conditioned yourself to a particular type of person that has become a "trigger group" for you. A trigger group is different than a mere preference for a particular characteristic of a woman. When you actually see someone with the particular characteristics from your trigger group, you may go into immediate objectifying of that person and shortly thereafter (almost unconsciously) fanta-size and reinforce it through ejaculation. For some addicts, a trigger group is a couple of very specific characteristics such as a woman with red hair and well built. For others, just one characteristic is their trigger group.

In some addict's addiction, they may be more predatory in nature and their trigger group may be someone who is vulnerable at the time, such as any drunk woman or maybe a woman with low self-esteem. Some trigger groups may be criminal in nature. The trigger group may also be prostitutes. Whatever the trigger group is for you, it is important to identify it in advance so that you can be alerted that this group is dangerous for your recovery. These trigger groups should be avoided at all costs early in your recovery. It probably is best to make a phone call if you chose to be around your trigger group or if it just happens, such as at work.

In the below space, describe your trigger group.

_____

_____

_____

_____

Who will I call if triggered?

1. _____

2. _____

3. _____

EXERCISE # 16

<u>WHERE NOT TO GO</u>

Sexual addiction and boundaries don't mix very well together. In your sexual acting-out days, you probably wouldn't be able to recognize a boundary if you tripped over one. In your sexual addiction freedom life-style, it will be very important for you to set some limitations for your own safety and recovery. Boundaries simply mean to establish some guidelines for places that you don't need to go to. As long as you stay within your boundaries, you can be safer from your addiction than if you don't have a conscious list of boundaries.

List below the places that you believe could hinder your freedom from sexual addiction. See the example.

<u>EXAMPLE</u>	<u>YOUR LIST</u>
1. <u>Adult Bookstore</u>	1. _____
2. <u>Adult Dance Hall</u>	2. _____
3. <u>Massage Parlor</u>	3. _____
4. <u>School Campus</u>	4. _____
5. <u>Beach/pool</u>	5. _____
	6. _____
	7. _____
	8. _____
	9. _____
	10. _____

The more cautious the list of boundaries in early recovery, the more it may keep you from slipping.

EXERCISE # 17

WHO I SHOULDN'T SEE

Talking about boundaries with someone else can be uncomfortable. Most people want to be liked by everybody. An addict, whether knowingly or unknowingly, surrounds himself many times with other addicts. This makes it tough, as you decide whom you shouldn't see during early recovery. You may ask, "Do I have to give up all my friends?" Hopefully not all your friends are linked to your sexual addiction although some may not be in your best interest to spend time with.

Setting boundaries around people you should not see may be necessary for the first 90 days only. For some people however, you truly do have to look at possibly ending those relationships. No friend is worth shame, guilt, lack of intimacy and staying addicted to sex, and no real friend would ask that of you. Remember, "how can two walk together unless they are agreed?" And "bad company corrupts good morals," Amos 3:3.

In considering boundaries around people you should not see, ask yourself the following questions.

1. Have I acted out with this person in a sexual way in the past?
2. Am I grooming this person for a sexual encounter?
3. Do I see this person more as an object or a person?
4. Does this person have pornography accessible if I visit them?
5. Do I think this person may be a sex addict?
6. Could I relapse around this person?
7. Does this person use sexual humor or talk about others as if they were objects?
8. Have I gone with this person to places on my "where not to go" boundary list.

Answering "yes" to one or more of these questions may make this person a risk to your recovery. With as much honesty as you can, try to fill in the columns below.

People I Know I Can't Be With	Try-and-See People	Safe People to Be With
1. _____	1. _____	1. _____
2. _____	2. _____	2. _____
3. _____	3. _____	3. _____
4. _____	4. _____	4. _____
5. _____	5. _____	5. _____

EXERCISE # 18

BOUNDARIES: ENTERTAINMENT

Television Boundaries

Television presents some real dilemmas for sex addicts. The current pop culture is a highly sexual one. The increase of sexually explicit scenes, jokes, innuendoes and the showing of naked bodies and extramarital activities on television and movie screens can trigger the sex addict into a myriad of sexual thoughts and behaviors. This doesn't even include the issues of the commercials that are often erotic, sexual, objectifying of women or the talk shows that usually concentrate on nonrecovering sex addicts. Remember that Lot "Vexed his righteous soul by seeing and hearing unrighteousness," II Peter 2:7-8. Vexed or tormented is exactly what can happen to the Christian sex addict who is exposed to sexual lewdness on television, especially cable television.

Television is not a safe place for sex addicts especially for the early part of their recovery. Here are some boundaries that many sex addicts in my practice have chosen in order to maintain a successful recovery.

1. No television at all for the first 90 days of recovery
2. Pre-selected television shows only
3. No channel surfing
4. Mute the commercials
5. No talk shows
6. No watching television alone
7. No television in the bedroom
8. Only watch television with family in the family room
9. No television past a certain time (10 P.M. or 11 P.M.)
10. No television in the middle of the night
11. No cable television within the first 90 days of recovery
12. No cable television at all
13. No pay-per-view television

In the following spaces, you may want to list your television boundaries for the next 90 days.

_____   _____

_____   _____

_____   _____

_____   _____

(Cont'd on next page)

If I relapse once due to a television experience I will _____.

If I relapse twice due to a television experience I will _____.

If I relapse three times due to a television experience I will _____.

The person I will be accountable to for my television boundaries and consequences is

_____.

I will check in on this issue with the above person ☐daily.   ☐weekly   ☐bimonthly.

Movie and Video Boundaries

Movies/videos are a dangerous place for sex addicts trying hard to recover successfully. The movie theater can be a nightmare if you don't have boundaries in place. I can't begin to tell you how many stories I have heard of precious freedom being damaged by a sex addict without pre-thought out movie boundaries.

Movies/videos are a great form of entertainment and can be enjoyed in a safe manner even for sex addicts. I myself enjoy movies, but like other successfully recovering addicts, only with firm boundaries. Some of the boundaries that sex addicts in my practice have utilized in order to maintain sobriety are as follows.

1. No movies within the first 90 days of recovery
2. No "X" or "R" rated movies
3. No "R" rated movies for the first 90 days of recovery
4. No "R" or "PG-13" rated movies (PG-13 can have full nudity)
5. Only go to movies that I would take a child to see ("PG" or "G" rated)
6. Read movie reviews in paper and avoid "nudity" or "adult situation" movies

Fill in the spaces below listing your movie/video boundaries.

My movie boundaries are:

_____   _____

_____   _____

_____   _____

If I relapse once due to a movie/video, I will _____.

(cont'd next page)

If I relapse twice due to a movie/video, I will _____.

If I relapse three times due to a movie/video, I will _____.

The person I will be accountable to for my movie/video boundaries is _____.

I will check in on my movie/video boundaries ❑daily. ❑weekly. ❑bi-monthly.

Magazine Boundaries

Being the visual creatures that many sex addicts are, magazines can stimulate them into unhealthy thoughts. Magazines have made objectifying women a science. Magazines are created to get you into a fantasy state so that you buy their products. The magazines I am talking about are pop magazines (not pornography store magazines—hopefully this is already a set boundary).

Magazines you may want to set a boundary with can also include catalogues such as *Victoria's Secret* (many sex addicts have lost sobriety here), whether it be a mailed magazine/catalogue or one purchased at a store. Be honest as far as the ones you can and cannot participate in if you are choosing to recover successfully. Your boundaries may change in the future as you get further in recovery, but let's fill in the below chart now.

Magazines I can read	Magazines I can't read	If relapse due to magazine, I will discontinue it
_____	_____	_____
_____	_____	_____
_____	_____	_____
_____	_____	_____
_____	_____	_____
_____	_____	_____
_____	_____	_____

(cont'd on next page)

Personal Advertisement Page

Some sex addicts have utilized professional services such as parlors, phone sex, lingerie modeling, and prostitutes from the personal advertisement page of the newspaper. Some sex addicts tempt themselves by "just talking" to these services. If these rituals are part of your addiction, you may consider these boundaries that have helped others get and maintain sobriety.

1. No newspaper reading for 90 days
2. Throw out entire classified section immediately.
3. Block all 900 number calls on your phone (this is a free service with some phone companies)
4. Get accountable to someone about this boundary

Fill in the following spaces to redefine your boundaries for personal advertisement viewing.

❑My personal advertising page boundary is _____.

❑If I relapse one time due to personal ads I will _____.

❑If I relapse two times due to personal ads I will _____.

❑If I relapse three times due to personal ads I will _____.

❑The person I am going to make myself accountable to for these boundaries is

_____.

EXERCISE # 19

BOUNDARIES: OBJECTS

Similar to alcoholism, sexual addiction has many different varieties of addicts. With alcohol, one may be a martini, brandy or beer alcoholic, however, all are alcoholics. With sexual addiction, you can have any number of behaviors and/or combinations of behaviors. Some sex addicts have included objects such as sex toys of one kind or another in their sexual acting out. Other sex addicts have issues about wearing particular clothes.

The need to have boundaries in this area is vital. It is important for sex to be relational with your wife and for you to move from conditioning yourself from objectifying sex to relational sex. If this issue applies to you, an honest discussion with your support person or therapist may be helpful to clarify your boundaries around sexual objects.

My boundaries with objects are:

1. _____

2. _____

3. _____

4. _____

EXERCISE # 20

<u>BOUNDARIES: BEING SEXUAL WITH MYSELF</u>

Masturbation is one of the areas in sexual addiction recovery that must be discussed and managed for a successful recovery. For most sex addicts, masturbation is the first sexual experience they were exposed to and it continued throughout early adolescence and young adulthood. Many sex addicts have hundreds if not thousands of hours of repeating the fantasy states compounded by masturbation. Some have created psychological, spiritual and/or biological dependence on this ritualistic sexual conditioning. It is for this reason masturbation must be taken very seriously. For most addicts, it is the foundation of their sexual addiction and remains a consistent reinforcement and can lead to reinforced fantasies. Reinforced fantasies lead to sexual behavior eventually.

It is my experience that the sex addict will seek out anything put into fantasies and then act it out if the fantasy is reinforced by masturbation. This may take one to two years but as one youth pastor said who currently is in jail for child molesting, "I didn't think I'd ever actually do it."

Because masturbation is such a foundational sexual behavior for most sex addicts, your goal is to move toward abstinence. In most cases, this will be a process. It is imperative that you keep your progress in sight and not focus on your failures. Condemnation over setbacks brings on hopelessness, which prevents you from accomplishing your goal.

Biblically, we are instructed to be self-controlled in <u>all</u> areas of life and to keep our thought life pure (1 Thes. 4:3-8, Gal. 5:22-24, Phil. 4:8, 2 Cor. 10:3-5). Right now, that may seem like a mountain too big to climb. Psalm 121:1 tells us to lift our eyes ABOVE the hills that stand against us and draw our strength from God. You CANNOT do this alone. You <u>will</u> be able to accomplish this feat through the power of the Holy Spirit and with the aid and support of others.

The Masturbation Checklist on page 35 will assist you in finding out what is motivating you to masturbate. By knowing your true motivations, you will be able to choose permanent solutions to your needs rather than the temporary "high" of masturbation.

EXERCISE # 21

MASTURBATION CHECK LIST

		YES	NO
1.	Am I trying to medicate a feeling?	____	____
2.	Am I confused about what I am feeling?	____	____
3.	Am I responding to a picture, movie or fantasy?	____	____
4.	Am I violating a boundary that I set for my recovery?	____	____
5.	Do I have a legitimate relational sexual outlet?	____	____
6.	Will I feel badly about myself afterwards?	____	____
7.	The last time I did this, did it send me on a binge of acting out?	____	____
8.	Will I want to keep this a secret?	____	____
9.	Am I using this as a stress release?	____	____

EXERCISE # 22

<u>LISTING MY BOUNDARIES</u>

Compiling a single list of all your boundaries can help you be aware of the different facets of your addiction. This list of boundaries may be a helpful reminder to review daily, or regularly, during your recovery. Your boundaries are already written out on previous pages. Just place in the spaces below a concise list of all of these boundaries.

<u>Boundaries where I can go.</u>

_____   _____

_____   _____

_____   _____

<u>Boundaries for who I can see.</u>

_____   _____

_____   _____

_____   _____

<u>Boundaries for objects.</u>

_____   _____

_____   _____

_____   _____

<u>Boundaries for the Internet.</u> (Exercise #26)

_____   _____

_____   _____

_____   _____

Boundaries for being sexual with myself. (If single)

_____   _____

_____   _____

_____   _____

Boundaries for television viewing

_____   _____

_____   _____

_____   _____

Boundaries for movies/videos.

_____   _____

_____   _____

_____   _____

Boundaries for personal advertisement pages.

_____   _____

_____   _____

_____   _____

EXERCISE # 23

BOUNDARIES ABOUT BOUNDARIES

In your recovery, you will go through many different stages. During your growth, you may consider moving your boundaries around. This can be a positive experience if the timing is right, or it can lead to a relapse and may be a premeditated step toward a trigger or acting-out.

In general, it is good to have some boundaries about boundaries. When changing your boundaries to be less restrictive you may want to include talking to your sponsor, pastor or therapist before you make a decision. Ask God about the change and wait for a week or month after you decide to move a boundary before you actually do it. Together these boundaries about boundaries are helpful to prevent you from arbitrarily changing them.

As an addict, you may be more likely to make a change because of a particular "feeling" instead of what may be in your best interest. Your addiction is very crafty at manipulating you through your emotions so it is best to have an external source that you can double check with to safeguard your precious recovery, especially during the first year of recovery.

Before changing a boundary, I will contact the following people.

1. _____

2. _____

3. _____

4. _____

EXERCISE # 24

SEXUAL BOUNDARIES

By now, you are probably getting the sense that recovery from sex addiction has something to do with identifying and maintaining boundaries. This is true of any recovery, whether it is alcohol, drugs, sex, or food. During your sexual addiction recovery, you will need to address the sex act itself and identify what is healthy for you and your wife.

The sexual history you may have had with your wife may be long and scarred by your addiction. I have worked with couples where the addict involved his wife in unwanted sexual behaviors. These events were traumatic for her. If these situations have occurred in your past, it may be necessary for you to consider providing her with professional help so that she can return to a healthy sexual relationship.

Boundaries involving the sex act need to be agreed upon by both partners, not just yourself. For most sex addicts, the growth in your sexuality will seem awkward at first but in the long run will increase the possibility of a great, mutually enjoyable sex life together. You and your wife may use the following checklist. Anything that doesn't have a "yes," (remember, no pressuring!) by her and you would constitute something you will not do during the sex act.

Sexual Behavior	Myself		My Wife	
_____	Y	N	Y	N
_____	Y	N	Y	N
_____	Y	N	Y	N
_____	Y	N	Y	N
_____	Y	N	Y	N
_____	Y	N	Y	N
_____	Y	N	Y	N
_____	Y	N	Y	N

(Cont'd on next page)

Our mutual boundaries are:

_____   _____

_____   _____

_____   _____

_____   _____

If I violate these boundaries, my consequences are:

1st time _____

2nd time_____

3rd time_____

Circle one:

I will make myself accountable to my ❑therapist.   ❑sponsor.   ❑other (same sex)_____.

EXERCISE # 25

SEXUAL BOUNDARIES FOR THE UNMARRIED

The single or divorced sex addict has to reestablish boundaries around his sexual behavior with others during recovery. The first of these boundaries might be "Who will I have sex with?" This may seem strange since in your acting-out days, you would rarely disqualify anyone from a sexual acting out experience. In recovery, the sex addict has learned that sex isn't about "getting something" but rather about "relationships." Some areas of concern as to whom you will have sex with are:

1. My wife/ex-wife
2. Past relationships or acting-out partners
3. Prostitutes
4. Someone I just met or someone I know less than a preset length of time
5. Someone I have no commitment toward
6. Someone who is married to someone else
7. Someone no more than 5 or so years younger than myself.

"When should I have sex?" Is a question few sex addicts have pondered during their sexual acting-out days. This question is also part of the boundary list you must develop as a recovering sex addict. Since sex is about a committed relationship, and biblically, sex outside of marriage is sin and will hurt you, a boundary is important to establish. This boundary may be something you will want to discuss with your group or support person.

"Why am I having sex?" is also a great recovering question to ask yourself <u>before</u> you have sex rather than afterward. Is a sexual relationship a commitment you are willing to make to this person? Most women (who are not sex addicts) believe sex has meaning and feel it is a form of commitment. God also shares this concept and wants you to have sex with only the one you are married to.

My sexual boundaries are:

_____

_____

_____

EXERCISE # 26

<u>THE INTERNET PROBLEM</u>

Sex addiction definitely keeps up with the technological advances of man. First there were drawings, then photographs, 8 mm, and videos and now we have CD ROMS, cyber-sex computer pornography and even virtual reality sex available. These new technologies can be highly addictive and isolating and they need to be addressed now for sex addicts.

The internet provides an outlet for sex addicts to access many of these technologies including pornography. The internet problem can be addressed in several approaches. Four are listed below.

1. There are Christian service providers that block out porn, chat rooms and news groups. I strongly encourage this. Most Christian radio stations can help you locate one. Focus on the Family in Colorado Springs also has a current list of Christian service providers and software blockers.
2. Software blockers are less effective but can be purchased at most software stores.
3. You can buy a key lock or a finger print lock as well at a computer store. (Let your wife have the key.)
4. You can remove the modem by taking it to a computer store.

My boundaries on the internet are:

- ❑ No internet availability
- ❑ Only when wife in the room (password protected or locked)
- ❑ Only with a protected service provider
- ❑ Other _____

NOTE: The internet does provide our home page for sex addiction product information at www.sexaddict.com

We offer two free e-mail newsletters: one for sex addicts and one for their wives.

EXERCISE # 27

REROUTING

Many sex addicts have particular driving routes that feed their sexual addiction. These routes may include driving by a certain convenience store, adult book store, adult dance club, billboard or massage parlor. Many of these places become a regular part of the sex addicts driving route. Before or after work or maybe on lunch break, the addict will go to one of several places to get a "look" and experience his addiction once again.

Conditioning yourself to these places is very powerful. Driving by any of the above places can often trigger you into thoughts of acting out or even rationalizations such as "I've had a bad day. I deserve this." Many sex addicts feel the rush their body receives by simply driving by an adult store or service. Some addicts even have to reroute the way they drive to work because of billboards that objectify women.

To reroute your driving is to carefully consider the way you go to or back from a geographical area. If you have a relapse because of your driving route, it definitely is an indication that rerouting has to happen. You can make rerouting a part of your accountability and that you won't drive by the school, pool or college campus or other possible relapse situations for your personal recovery. Rerouting can help stop some of the ritual acting-out of driving by the old familiar place where you have acted-out so many times in the past.

Rerouting can also be applied to those who work in offices where a particular female sex addict or victim is working that we have objectified in the past. Find ways not to walk the route past their desk or office. If it is a waitress, you can choose to eat at another restaurant. The quicker you can reroute your life, the easier it will be for your recovery.

EXERCISE # 28

<u>DEFENSIVE DRIVING</u>

As a general rule, sex addicts have the ability to disconnect from themselves, especially while driving. Another word that clinicians use for the word *disconnecting* is "disassociating" from oneself. Disassociating is what the addict does right before he starts going into a fantasy.

Driving is very conducive to getting into a disconnected or disassociated state. This is probably because of the routine of driving. The limited amount of concentration it takes to drive, and the sheer repetition of most places you drive to, demands little from your brain so you can think about other things.

This is where the sex addict often starts planting the seeds for his next victim or "adventure." The sex addict needs a plan to drive defensively. Some tips other addicts have been successful with are:

1. Utilize the rubber band technique while driving.
2. Listen to talk radio instead of music - this engages your thoughts more than a song you may have heard hundreds of times. You are also less likely to hit a song that may remind you of some event or person.
3. Listen to books on tape or recovery tapes.
4. When you see someone of the opposite sex, look to the opposite side of the road until you pass them and then count to ten before you look back so you resist the "rear view mirror glance."
5. When coming up to a light with someone from the opposite sex or your trigger group in the car next to you, keep your eyes on the driver's license plate ahead of you.
6. When passing someone of the opposite sex or trigger group (that you want to look at) keep your eyes on an object ahead of you.
7. Once you know where the billboards are that are sexual or that are advertising adult places, practice driving by or looking at the other side of the road.

Practicing these tips may help driving experiences be less of a threat to your journey toward freedom. Some who are concerned about their driver safety say they can't do these casually. Let me point out that an addict with neck turning or stretching abilities, is a threat to themselves and those around him. Driving defensively can keep you from beginning your addictive thoughts, which can lead to a more successful recovery not to mention a safer drive!

EXERCISE # 29

ACCOUNTABILITY: TIME

Sex addicts who want to act out have to find time to do so. This time they *find* may be used to groom or "romance" someone, to cruise, get pornography or simply to just get alone for a little while. Since a sex addict has a secret life and doesn't tell anyone what behaviors he is up to, he has to develop a few escape patterns.

The first pattern is to lie about where he was and what he was doing. The second pattern that the addict develops is a lifestyle (including his job) that has wide open gaps of unaccountable time. Some favorite vocations for sex addicts appear to be salespeople (of all types), doctors, lawyers, self-employed and other mobile jobs that keep them unaccountable and unavailable for their time. This lifestyle makes it much easier for them to "slip out" so they can act-out without anyone questioning them. The sex addict doesn't even have to lie directly. This is not to say that those who have 9-5 jobs or who stay in one location are less likely to be a sex addict. Sex addicts in 9-5 jobs may develop "hobbies" or "social outlets" such as softball that can leave blank spaces of time so that they can be unaccountable for their acting-out activities.

The point is that acting-out takes unaccountable time, so the reverse is true about getting into recovery. Getting freedom for a sex addict means being accountable with your time with someone of the same sex. This would exclude your spouse, but may be your sponsor, someone else in the program or a friend who is aware of your situation and who will go over your schedule with you. This will help you not get that "Oh, I'm alone and nobody knows" feeling which is very familiar to sex addicts and dangerous to a recovering sex addict.

EXERCISE # 30

ACCOUNTABILITY: MONEY

Being accountable for finances has saved many sex addicts from acting-out and losing their precious freedom. This technique can stop many forms of acting-out instantly. For many sex addicts, most acting-out behaviors take money. Money is what makes the very sick illicit sexual world go around. Without money, even in the addict's most desperate emotional state, he can not purchase anything. Simply put, accountability with money can save your sobriety.

How this can be practiced will probably be an individual matter. The following are some methods for financial accountability that have helped some sex addicts in their recovery.

1. Go strictly to credit card spending only and review statements with wife or support person at the end of the month
2. Review gas credit card bills to check that the gas station you are going to does not regularly have pornography accessible.
3. Use checks only and review them monthly with support person
4. Allow your spouse to fully know about finances
5. Have spouse or support person fully aware of secret stashes of money, odd jobs, or free-lance work that you do and how much you earn.

Once you get committed to the concept of being financially accountable and how it may be in your best interest for the first 6-12 months of your recovery, you will find a way to make money accountability work for you. I find that when the creativity of an addict is working on how to make their recovery a priority, there is a lot of hope for their recovery. The addict, who makes excuses and looks for ways that he can not be accountable financially, is probably going to experience relapses that involve money in his acting-out. This can be prevented by financial accountability.

Remember that sexual addiction recovery is probably going to be the hardest undertaking of your life. You must be willing to go to any length. For most, this may mean initially becoming financially accountable to someone. This technique can get to the bare roots of your acting-out. My hope is that those reading this exercise can take this step into a life of freedom from sexual addiction.

EXERCISE # 31

STEP ONE

*"We admitted that we were powerless over our sexual addiction
and that our lives had become unmanageable."*

This is the most important step of all. In Step One, you place your feet on the path toward freedom. "We" means that you will have others involved with you in your recovery. Recovery is a team participation sport. "We admitted" is not all of Step One. Some people attend meetings and never complete Step One. Some simply admit they are a sex addict much like the alcoholic admits he is an alcoholic while drinking a beer.

Step One has us admit that we are "powerless." Powerlessness is different than being addicted. Being addicted to cocaine could mean that if you saw some cocaine, "you couldn't help yourself" and you would use the cocaine. Powerlessness would be if you saw the cocaine, you would run out and call someone, and try any helpful behaviors to avoid what once controlled your life.

Many lives are tainted with the unmanageability that sex addiction brings. In your recovery, sanity and order will replace the "crazies" and the chaos. Step One is the beginning to a life-style of freedom from sexual addiction. In the workbook, *Steps to Freedom*, I provide over 20 pages that allow you to explore and experience Step One. This is how important I feel Step One is.

Behaviors that support Step One are:

BEHAVIOR		YES	NO
1.	Prayer	____	____
2.	Reading	____	____
3.	Phone calls	____	____
4.	Meetings	____	____
5.	Staying accountable with your time and money	____	____
6.	Creativity in your recovery	____	____

EXERCISE # 32

90 MEETINGS IN 90 DAYS

"Ninety meetings in ninety days" is an old Alcoholics Anonymous saying. What it meant was that an alcoholic starting recovery was asked to attend an AA meeting every day. This behavior provided several benefits: 1) It allowed the alcoholic to see recovery in other's lives, and gave hope for recovery, 2) It enabled the alcoholic to hear what it meant to be honest about life, 3) It gave the alcoholic a new group of people to call friends and, 4) It helped the addict receive support for struggles and gain recognition for efforts made to stay clean.

This tool works. Going to that many meetings up front will guarantee a change in your life. Unfortunately, only in the very large cities would there be a possibility of this many meetings happening in the sex anonymous groups. The principle is true. Wherever you live, find the local sex recovery groups and go to as many groups as possible for the first 90 days. It can help build the relationships you need to get and stay free.

Sex addiction recovery is a team sport; you can't do it by yourself. The group will help you become successful in your recovery. Again, if you feel like starting a Freedom Group (a Christ-based 12-Step support group) talk to your pastor. According to one of our studies of pastors across 7 denominations with 14 years in the ministry, **84%** stated they would welcome such a group in their church if a church member approached them and the church member would lead the group.

EXERCISE # 33

USING CHECK-IN TIMES

Unlike Alcoholics Anonymous which has only one support group available, in the sex addiction recovery movement, there are several different support groups you can go to. The 12 Step support groups vary in names (see appendix) and in practices. To make it even more complicated these groups vary from state to state.

Check-in time is something that is common in all 12 Step meetings. The check-in time is usually held at the end of the support group meeting. The larger group who wishes to utilize check-in times, breaks off into smaller groups of 2 or 3 people. This is where you get "current" or honest about where you are for that day.

If there have been fantasies or behaviors that you have been involved in with your sex addiction, the check-in time is where you would get honest about it. Check-ins has saved many addicts from acting out behaviors. This level of honesty can only keep you closer to your goal of recovery. If your group does not employ a check in-time, you can start this with one other person so you can gain the benefit of this exercise.

In the early part of your recovery, make sure you check-in at every meeting you go to. This will save you some struggles with your addiction and make your recovery go much smoother. This will also keep you from getting lulled into a false sense of recovery by "just attending meetings." If all you do is attend meetings and are not using this time for personal honesty, you will struggle much more in your attempt to get free. Remember maximized thinking. Give as much of yourself as you can during check-ins and you will not regret it.

EXERCISE # 34

<u>MY SPONSOR</u>

A sponsor in a 12-step group is similar to a mentor or a discipleship relationship. The sponsor can be someone who has been where you are and knows how to get further in sexual freedom than you. A good sponsor would be someone you could call regularly and talk to about recovery. A sponsor will encourage you to do your step work and help hold you account-able to goals you have set for yourself in recovery.

In picking a sponsor, you probably want to listen to others in your support group who are really in recovery. This would probably be someone who isn't reporting the latest relapse story but rather is working the steps. It is best if this person has finished his fifth step. This eliminates your sponsor from helping you through while dealing with his own garbage. After the fifth step, there is a lot less shame and someone can be much healthier to help you.

Some sex addicts like to have a sponsor who has at least six months in the program or six months of freedom from bottom line behaviors. This would be ideal. The reality is that sex addict support groups in some areas are just starting, and most of the members will not have that kind of sobriety.

Utilizing a sponsor relationship can help tremendously to not feel alone during your recovery. This healthy relationship hopefully will allow you to see that there is more in recov-ery for you in the future. Ask the person you are considering to be your sponsor what a good time would be to talk together about sponsoring you. If you mutually agree, this would be your sponsor.

EXERCISE # 35

IDENTIFYING & COMMUNICATING FEELINGS

Most addicts have difficulty with identifying feelings. If an addict (of any kind) has a feeling, he generally fixes it by taking a drink, drug, sex or some other way of medicating this feeling.

Most sex addicts have not had any experience from their family of origin in the area of how to have and share feelings. Feelings are a skill that you can develop and acquire levels of mastery once you have practiced.   This can be related to growing up and not learning how to maintain a car. It doesn't mean that you are less intelligent or worthwhile because you can't fix a car. You would be simply untrained. If you were to take a class on car maintenance, you would probably be a good mechanic. The difference is that the skills you are exposed to and have learned will make you more skilled.

Expressing feelings, in sexual addiction recovery, is very important for several reasons. Some are mentioned below.

1.   In your acting-out days, if you had a feeling, you probably would not know what it was. But if you masturbated or acted out in some way, the feeling would go away. In this process, you may not have learned to identify feelings and hence can not meet your own real needs.

2.   In your early recovery, between usually the third to sixth week of abstinence from your acting out behaviors, (including masturbation for most sex addicts) you may begin to start recognizing feelings. This feels almost like a thawing out of emotions. It is best to have already begun to identify your feelings so that they don't confuse or overwhelm you and activate the cycle (feel —> act out —> feeling disappears). In recovery, you get to feel without acting-out.

3.   As a relapse prevention, if you can identify your feelings, you may better know how to handle or manage these feelings in order to prevent relapses.

4.   If a cycle or relapse occurs, you may be able to track down what emotion(s) preceded this and move forward in your recovery process.

5.   Mastering your feelings can allow more intimacy into your life and yes, it will make your sex life better, too.

In the first month or so of your recovery, the feelings identification exercise may be one of the harder exercises in this book. The discipline you put into this exercise will have lifelong benefits in every area of your life including relationships, parenting, work, recovery, spirituality, and your social life. It may also save you from financial mistakes because your intuition will become more active in your decision making process.

(Cont'd next page)

The feelings exercise is simple. Fill in the blanks. An example is given below.

1.   I feel <u>(feeling word)</u> when _____. (Present tense)
2.   I first remember feeling <u>(same feeling word)</u> when _____. (Past tense)

EXAMPLE:

1.   I feel <u>Calm</u> when <u>I am on the lake in a boat with a friend.</u>
2.   I first remember feeling <u>calm</u> when <u>I was 10 years old, I had my own bedroom where I played with a race car set.</u>

The goal here is to have two experiences. In computer terms, an addict has an emotional database, but this database has no file names so you can't access the files nor can you utilize this data. This exercise, if you do two or more daily for a month to six weeks, will make your journey toward freedom a lot smoother. Those who do this in their recovery early, never regret it later. Those who don't do this exercise, always regret it. So, I strongly encourage you to take the time to do this exercise today and for the next several weeks.

A list of feelings that you can utilize for your feeling exercises is located in the Appendix of this book. The list is in alphabetical order. You can pick out whatever feeling you want to practice randomly from the feelings list.

FEELINGS COMMUNICATION

When you have ten or more of your feelings identified, it is important that you begin to communicate them to a safe person. A safe person in your recovery group or a person who you are accountable to can be helpful at this. The person's role is simply to listen, not really give feedback. If you choose your spouse, make sure this is safe for you and **make sure your examples do not involve your spouse in any way.**

If you involve your spouse, she can do the exercise and identify and communicate feelings back to you also. This can be a great opportunity to develop intimacy. If these experiences turn into disagreements, the exercise is being done wrong and you may need to pick another person or a therapist to do them with.

When sharing your feelings, it is important to maintain eye contact with the person you are sharing them with. This eye contact with a person may feel uncomfortable at first, but will eventually be comfortable to you. This is part of the benefit of this exercise. If you do them with your spouse there is to be no discussion of what was shared in this exercise until 72 hours after the feeling was shared.

EXERCISE # 36

<u>DANGEROUS "E" ZONES</u>

Emotions for sex addicts can be tricky. Many sex addicts early in recovery have few feeling skills. During your recovery, especially after completing your feeling exercises, you will become better acquainted with yourself and your feelings.

Being aware of your feelings will be helpful, but it will not make them less difficult. In your recovery journey, you will find that some feelings are very difficult for you to manage. Some feelings may include but are not limited to the feelings: *bored, lonely, angry, hopeless, worthless, shame and rejection.*

These difficult feelings are what I call the dangerous "E" zones. They are feelings that you have skillfully avoided or medicated during your addiction. Often these feelings in reverse are what you received from your addiction: active, connected, content, hopeful, esteemed, shameless and fully accepted. This is what makes these feelings a possible dangerous "E" zone. They represent a cluster of feelings that you rarely felt without your addiction.

During your recovery, you need to find out what your dangerous "E" zones are. The easiest way is to take the feeling list and put a mark by those feelings you believe to be most difficult for you. List these feeling words below.

_____

_____

_____

EXERCISE # 37

ACTION PLANS FOR MY FEELINGS

In the previous exercise, you listed the feelings that could be your dangerous "E" zones. In this exercise, you will take the time to give yourself several options if you get into one of these zones. Having a written plan ahead of time helps a lot in recovery. This exercise will be a greater help if you can practice and hold the feeling for 15 seconds and then implement a plan of your choice. This practice will help when the real battle is on.

The following is an example to practice.

I feel <u>bored</u>. Hold this <u>bored</u> feeling 15-30 seconds. Call someone in the program.

Below list the feelings that are dangerous "E" zones for you and list three behavioral options for that feeling.

EXAMPLE:

Feeling: <u>Bored</u>

1. Call someone
2. Go to a meeting
3. Exercise

Feeling: _____

1. _____
2. _____
3. _____

Feeling: _____

1. _____
2. _____
3. _____

Feeling: _____

1. _____
2. _____
3. _____

EXERCISE # 38

AVOID H.A.L.T.

During the recovery process whether it is for alcohol, drugs, sex or food, *H.A.L.T.* has been used in support group settings to stand for <u>H</u>ungry, <u>A</u>ngry, <u>L</u>onely and <u>T</u>ired. These are important things to avoid for the recovering sex addict as well. Simply put, keep yourself eating regularly and properly not allowing yourself to get too hungry which may make your more susceptible to less logical thinking. Some researchers believe that eating certain foods can help you in recovery. A book that discusses this aspect of recovery is *Help Yourself*, by Joel Robertson and published by Thomas Nelson Publishing.

Anger can sneak up on you quickly and put you in an emotional state of "I'll show you" and you could begin to rationalize why it might be okay to act-out. Some sex addicts have a whole system where they purposely start a fight with their wife, leave, act-out and come back later justifying their acting-out behavior because they were "<u>A</u>ngry." Anger can be an important piece of managing your recovery.

<u>L</u>onely is a difficult feeling for the sex addict to handle. Feeling alone can make the sex addict vulnerable to want to medicate by acting-out. Having an action plan or an "I will do" list available in your wallet for when you get lonely may be helpful. Some other suggestions are:

1.   Go to a public place such as a mall, restaurant, etc.

2.   Call someone in the program.

3.   Plan ahead to avoid your alone time gaps such as weekends or when your wife may be out of town.

4.   Exercise

5.   Help someone else with a project

6.   Go to a meeting, church or other social gathering

7.   Pray

8.   Ask others what they do.

(Cont'd on next page)

Being "**T**ired" in your busy, fast paced life, is a familiar feeling. Tiredness can lower your resistance to the point of "who cares." To recover, we need to stay alert. Our sex addiction is a default program that wants to be fully activated anytime it can find a way to. To prevent tiredness, get regular sleep and if you need a rest here or there, take it if you can. List your action plan for the following.

Hungry - _____

_____

Angry - _____

_____

Lonely - _____

_____

Tired - _____

_____

EXERCISE # 39

<u>MY WORST MOMENT</u>

In the addict's active sexually addicted life-style, he rarely thinks of the pain he is causing himself or anyone else. In recovery from sex addiction, when the addiction "talks to you" it will try to sell you as to how "A little bit won't hurt," or "Who will know?" "You can act out just one more time." "You are sober enough." "It won't affect your recovery." These and many other lies try to maximize the current benefit your addiction will give to you (i.e. it feels good) and minimize the long term effects (i.e. this could be the beginning of two-to-ten year binge and you could lose your marriage, business and quite possibly get a sexually transmitted disease). This addiction is very crafty!

A tool that has helped recovering addicts maintain recovery is having a negative experience locked in, almost memorized that maximizes the pain and minimizes the pleasure to act out. For some sex addicts this picture could include the possibility of getting caught by the police. For others, their worst picture is getting kicked out of the house for good, seeing their child's faces when they leave, seeing their spouse cry, hearing a judge say "no visitation privileges," the loss of a job, risking AIDS or even abortions. These are only a few experiences. You may have one or more painful moments. You may want to write down these experiences to remind yourself.

After you write down these experiences, picture it in your mind as vividly as you can and feel the feelings. Practice this picture in a public place (you're not as likely to act out) 2 to 3 times a day for three days. Rehearsing this image and feeling will make you ready to beat the addiction when it starts talking to you.

The days I practiced this painful experience were:

1. _____

2. _____

3. _____

EXERCISE # 40

<u>WHAT MY ADDICTION COST ME</u>

Every addiction costs the addict something. You can talk about emotional, relational, social and vocational losses that occurred due to your sexual addiction all day. Although these are all important there is a practical side to the addict. The cost, in financial terms has helped some addicts put in perspective once again the damage that their sexual addiction has done to their life.

The knowledge of estimated financial damage has helped some addicts say "no" to acting out. When clients have done this exercise in my office, the average cost over the life-time of the addict to the point when they began recovery was approximately $250,000 dollars. Most of us wish we had that amount on hand today. To list the cost of your addiction, you may want to consider several things:

Time Value of your addiction (See Appendix B)   _____
Cost of actual pornographic material purchased   _____
Cost of professional sex services   _____
Cost of legal fees (including divorce)   _____
Divorce losses   _____
Child support   _____
Missed opportunities (college, job promotions)   _____
Working in a job below your abilities   _____
Loss of creativity and energy over years   _____
Guilt spending (spend to make you or wife feel better)   _____
Geographical moves (running from addiction)   _____
Emotional/financial immature choices due to addiction   _____
Other _____   _____
Other _____   _____
Other _____   _____

TOTAL   _____

When you see a person you want to objectify or act out with, some have found it helpful to take the total cost of what their addiction has cost them and visually place it over that person's head such as a cartoon caption. It's a great motivator for recovery.

EXERCISE # 41

COST CARD

In other exercises in this book such as *What My Addiction Took From Me*, *What My Addiction Cost Me*, and *My Worst Moment*, you may have discovered in several dimensions what sexual addiction has really cost you. This realization can truly be painful and you can have very sad feelings accompanying this realization.

Although at the moment you do feel this pain and discomfort, there will also be days ahead when your addiction will attempt to have you forget this moment. If your addiction can get you to forget this pain and discomfort, it will be easier to talk you into "another ride" on the sexual addiction train. It is in the pain and discomfort of what your addiction has cost you that will help you not to do it again. In the hopes of strengthening your recovery and giving you one more tool to recover by, you can capture this moment of pain to rescue yourself in the future days when your sex addiction wants you to join in again and destroy you.

Use the back of a business card that is blank and write at the top of it the word "COST" along with what your addiction has cost you and what it could cost you five years from now. Write yourself some notes that only you would understand and place it in your billfold. When you start to feel the addiction talk you into acting-out, pull out your card and talk back. Having the facts puts truth on your side and you may escape a relapse this time.

EXAMPLE:

COST

Now: $52,000
5 years: $135,000
When left house
Emotional illiterate
1 marriage

EXERCISE # 42

REWARD CARD

The reward card is very similar to the cost card. Actually it is the flip side of the cost card. Take a business card and on the backside, place some of the rewards you see for yourself such as your family and job if you maintain a successful recovery from sexual addiction. Be as specific as possible in your rewards such as staying married, seeing my children grow up, probably making more money and better sex.

Place these rewards on the backside of this business card so that you can clearly understand it at a quick glance. Some have found it helpful to tape the two cards together with *rewards* and *cost* easily read so in the "heat of the battle" so to speak with your addiction, you have both the pain of the past and the hope of the future to fight with. This two-edged sword can help you with one battle at a time.

If this tool helps you win the battle of sexual addiction just one time, it is worth keeping in your wallet or billfold for at least the first year of your freedom from sexual addiction.

EXERCISE # 43

<u>CALLING CARD</u>

In recovery as we discussed earlier, a phone call may be your only link to reality. In a moment, the addiction can sweep you off your feet and have you swirling in thoughts, pictures, devices and an entire host of feelings. It is as if you fell off a boat and it is moving away leaving you in a storm. Somehow you need to connect to the boat so someone, anyone, can throw you a life preserver to save your life.

In the case of the sex addiction storm, you can pull out your phone card, call someone and be pulled safely to the shore of recovery from the waters of sexual addiction. If you were left to yourself, you may have drown this time.

Simply put, keep phone numbers in your wallet, car, home and your office so at any place and anytime you can call someone when you feel the storm coming or while it may be in full swing so you don't have to experience a relapse that day. Remember you don't recover by yourself. It is much better to call first than to relapse and have to call later. The calling card is one tool that can save you in a difficult situation. So make your card as soon as possible.

The day I made my calling card _____.

EXERCISE # 44

<u>TURNING "IT" OVER</u>

This exercise is helpful to the recovering sex addict to lessen the need to be totally in control of your sexual organs. At some point in your recovery, you will do a Step Three. This is where you turn your "life and will" over to the care of God as you understand Him.

This decision includes your sexuality and sexual organs. Turning the decision of who you share your sexuality with including yourself doesn't have to be yours totally to make. You can turn your sexuality over to God and it can be freeing. As one addict stated "the way I figure, I'm the third person on the totem pole when it comes to my sexual organ. First is God, He made me, second is my spouse, and third is myself. If I can get my spouse and God's permission, I'm okay. If not, I'm not the sole owner."

This discussion may seem light but the results were life changing when this addict no longer felt responsible for his sexual organ. "That's God's business." The prayer is simple. Find a quiet time with God and communicate to Him that you are surrendering your sexual organ to do His will and not your own and that you will trust Him to manage it from here on out.

This prayer when internalized, can be an honest tool for recovery. Some make this a daily prayer in their early journey toward freedom from sexual addiction.

The day I said this prayer. _____

EXERCISE # 45

RELAPSE AND RESEARCH

Relapses in the very beginning may occur. Turning a relapse into research is very important to keep you from making the exact same mistake again. Researching your relapse takes rigorous honesty.

If you relapse, ask yourself the following questions.

❑ What were my feelings prior to acting-out?

❑ What red flags did I pass up?

❑ What tools in my recovery did I choose not to use?

❑ How many days have I been planning this event?

❑ Relapsing takes time, energy and sometimes money. What was the significance or importance to this acting-out event?

❑ At what point did I begin to feel "powerful" over my addiction?

❑ Have I regularly kept the Five Commandments prior to acting-out?

❑ What have I learned about myself in this relapse?

❑ What have I learned about my addiction?

❑ What needs to be different so I don't relapse this way again?

❑ Do I have to change some boundaries to stay free from sexual addiction?

The date I shared this with my support person _____.

The date I shared this with my support group _____.

EXERCISE # 46

<u>TRAVEL TIPS</u>

In today's world, it is not uncommon to go on business trips out of town or even out of the state or country. For some sex addicts this was their prime acting-out time. Unaccountable time and money make a dangerous combination for your addiction that wants to flare up, even in your recovery.

The following are traveling tips that have been used by those who have been successful in their sex addiction recovery.

1. If you travel a lot, get an SAA National Directory (or other sexual addiction support group listed in appendix) and find the meetings at that location a week in advance. You can get this also through our LINKS button on our website at www.sexaddict.com.

2. Call the sexual addiction meeting in the city you are visiting and make a breakfast, lunch or dinner appointment so that you know you'll be talking recovery with some one while on your trip.

3. Call your hotel before you leave and cancel all adult channels and/or pay for view television.

4. Take two rubber bands with you. One to put on your wrist to keep you from fantasy, the second to place around the armoire door knobs that carry the television to keep you from watching it "unintentionally."

5. Make at least daily phone calls to people in your home group and schedule these before you leave.

6. Take at least one sex addiction recovery book or workbook. <u>Steps to Freedom</u> or this book would be great choices.

7. When lonely, go to a public area in the hotel.

8. Keep the Five Commandments as much as possible while traveling.

9. Practice the *Turning it Over Prayer*.

PART TWO:

PERSONAL GROWTH FREEDOM TECHNIQUES

EXERCISE # 47

STEP TWO

"Came to believe a power greater than ourselves could restore us to sanity."

Coming to believe in one power that is able to heal you is a process. As Christians, we know this power is Jesus Christ. So did the writer of the Twelve Steps. The first writing of the Twelve Steps used the word "*God*" in place of "*power greater than ourselves.*" In the 1930's, they didn't think our culture would broaden this to anything else. In current traditional Twelve Step groups (not Freedom Groups), they take this step too loosely, but in Step Three, they continue with the word "God." Remember, believing is behaving. "If you love me, you will keep my commandments," John 14:15. Some sex addicts have so much shame about what they've done and who they have hurt, that they may feel defective.

In Step Two, if you have a religious background, this may be a place for you to rediscover a forgotten heritage. For others you will start with a totally clean slate spiritually and get the joy of discovering for the first time a connecting with Jesus Christ. A more thorough exploration of Step Two is given in the Steps to Freedom workbook made available in the back of this book.

Behaviors that support Step Two are:

BEHAVIOR		YES	NO
1.	Honesty about your spiritual place	_____	_____
2.	Prayer	_____	_____
3.	Meditation	_____	_____
4.	Biblical reading	_____	_____
5.	Dialoguing with others you feel have a good relationship with Jesus.	_____	_____

EXERCISE # 48

WHAT MY ADDICTION GAVE ME

When you think about a relationship as long as you have had with your addiction which may be 10, 20, 30 or more years, you have had quite a relationship. You ran to your addiction to celebrate, be encouraged, feel wanted, powerful, in control, confident and sexual on a regular basis. For most sex addicts, their sexual addiction was the only committed relationship they kept over the years.

Your addiction has given many things to you including, 1) a false world, 2) it kept your secret(s), 3) false intimacy, 4) a sense of success, 5) a totally unconditional loving relationship regardless of your deviancy, 6) acceptance, and the list goes on. In thinking about this, you must realize that you got a lot out of your addiction. If you didn't, you would have stopped a long time ago. In light of this, because each of you received different things out of your relationship with your sexual addiction. It is important in your recovery that you know what it was that you received from your addiction.

Make a real honest effort to list as many of the things as you can that you have received from your addiction. You can probably come up with twenty things that your addiction gave to you.

1. _____
2. _____
3. _____
4. _____
5. _____
6. _____
7. _____
8. _____
9. _____
10. _____
11. _____
12. _____
13. _____
14. _____
15. _____
16. _____
17. _____
18. _____
19. _____
20. _____

EXERCISE # 49

THANK YOU LETTER

In completing the previous exercise of listing the good things your sex addiction has done for you, the realization of how powerful, intimate and dynamic of a relationship you had with your sexual addiction is obvious. Write a thank you letter to your sexual addiction for all of the things it has done for you. This will crystallize further how, through the relationship with your sexual addiction, you were getting your needs met and had many years of devoted (although ultimately destructive) service toward you. You may need to use an additional piece of paper for this exercise.

To my sexual addiction,

_____

_____

_____

_____

_____

_____

_____

_____

_____

_____

_____

EXERCISE # 50

<u>WHAT MY ADDICTION TOOK FROM ME</u>

For every relationship, a list can be made of what losses and what gains come from it. Within a sexual addictive relationship, the list of what this relationship took from me was usually equal to or greater than the list of what that relationship temporarily gave to me. No where is this more true than with addiction.

My sexual addiction had stolen many years of my life and emotions. It had taken my ability to communicate due to the shame, guilt and fear of being exposed. I felt isolated and less than. I was scared about my secrets and feared never being truly loved. I was glassed in and couldn't feel a way out. I had a sense I was going nowhere. The list could go on and on such as "Will I ever be normal again?" or "Can God still love me?" We each have our own list of what addiction has taken from us. It is important in your freedom to look at these losses honestly. In the following spaces, list your losses that your sexual addiction has caused.

1. _____

2. _____

3. _____

4. _____

5. _____

6. _____

7. _____

8. _____

9. _____

10. _____

11. _____

12. _____

13. _____

14. _____

15. _____

16. _____

17. _____

18. _____

19. _____

20. _____

21. _____

22. _____

23. _____

24. _____

25. _____

26. _____

27. _____

28. _____

29. _____

30. _____

EXERCISE # 51

GOOD-BYE LETTER

There is a time of reckoning for every bad relationship and a time when you have to confront the relationship and say, this is not working for me. Many have had to do this with several unhealthy relationships. Some have had to go through the divorce process.

It is now that time for your relationship with your addiction. You can see by your list of what has been taken from you that you can no longer continue in such a harmful relationship. You must confront your addiction face to face, so to speak, and say good-bye to it. Your addiction isn't worth the past damage or the guaranteed progressive damage that it can cause. There is a saying: "a mind is a terrible thing to waste" and in the sex addict's case, it is your soul that is a terrible thing to waste.

During this sobering moment in your life, no matter how difficult, you must say good-bye to your relationship with your sexual addiction. In the space below, write a good-bye letter to your addiction.

Dear Sex Addiction,

_____

_____

_____

_____

_____

_____

_____

_____

_____

_____

EXERCISE # 52

<u>EMPTY CHAIR</u>

The "empty chair" exercise has helped many clients in therapy to not only experience but further the work they have completed in the previous exercises. The deeper you confront your sex addiction, the better sense of resolve you will experience. The sense of resolve you experience may be the one tool on any given day that may help you stay clean for the day.

In this exercise, you will sit in a chair and place another chair directly in front of you. Have your thank you and good-bye letters to your addiction with you while sitting in the chair. Read your letters out loud (no one else needs to be there unless you want support from a therapist) as if the sex addiction was a real person sitting in the chair in front of you. For most of your life the sex addiction was a real person. The experiences addicts have had with this exercise vary. In the space below, you can list your thoughts and feelings about this exercise.

My thoughts are:

_____

_____

_____

My feelings are:

_____

_____

_____

The date I completed this exercise: _____.

EXERCISE # 53

GRIEF STAGES

Sexual addiction has probably been your best friend and may seem like your only true friend. Quite possibly it has been there faithfully since adolescence. It has nurtured you, told you that you were special, worthwhile and sexual. It has accepted you no matter what hurts you brought into it or what kind of mood you were in that day. To choose recovery is to divorce yourself from this almost daily relationship which may know more about you than anyone else.

When you truly divorce yourself from your addiction, you will go through a grieving process. This process is normal and healthy. This exercise is to help expose you to the understanding of the stages of grief so that you can identify what stage you find yourself in and what stages you may have ahead of you.

SHOCK - This is the moment you realized that you really were a sex addict. Numbness or a sense of emotional nausea may accompany this. This stage is usually fleeting but may last minutes, hours, or sometimes days.

DENIAL - This stage can last for years. "I'm not the one with the problem, you are" is a comment some addicts in denial will say to their wives. "It's normal to do this." "This isn't sick, you are just naive." These statements and a thousand other statements like them are evidence of denial. Basically, if you are in denial, you "don't have a problem."

ANGER - This is the first stage in which you begin to process that you "may" be a sex addict. You are probably very angry at this realization. "Why me?" "Why can't I masturbate or act out in my own way? Other people can." You may dislike that you are an addict intensely, but at least you are finally wrestling with the painful truth of being an addict. This stage is often accompanied by mood swings, irritability and irrational behavior.

BARGAINING - This is the stage that someone might say, "I'm not an addict if..." The "if" can be "if I can stop for a while..." or "if I can just stop one aspect of my behavior." The addict may wish that "my wife was more sexual" then I would not have this problem. Bargaining seeks to relieve the sting of the fact that you may be a sex addict. This is a very creative stage.

SORROW - This is when it starts hitting you. You are a sex addict. This may not feel very good but it is true. You know that there are going to have to be changes. You can feel it. You are sad about the fact of being a sex addict and maybe what it has done to your life and the lives of those you tried to love.

ACCEPTANCE - "I am a sex addict." You now accept responsibility for your addiction. You are no longer blaming or looking for a magical way to avoid the process of recovery. Your behavior is active in recovery. Your creativity is being used to find time and ways to recover, and you are being honest even when it hurts to be.

In the space below, circle the stage that you believe you are currently in. In a few weeks, check back and see if there is movement. Grief is a process. Being in Grief is okay because if you pass denial, you are actively going through the reality of being a sex addict. You can also write about each stage you have experienced it.

❏SHOCK ❏DENIAL ❏ANGER ❏BARGAINING ❏SORROW ❏ACCEPTANCE

Shock _____

_____

Denial _____

_____

Anger _____

_____

Bargaining _____

_____

Sorrow _____

_____

Acceptance _____

_____

EXERCISE # 54

MEETING MY NEEDS

After you have completed the feeling exercise for about a month, you will have become more skilled at knowing what your feelings are. The skill of knowing your feelings is a necessary prerequisite to being able to meet your needs.

In your addiction in the past, if you had a feeling, you rarely knew what it was. But, if you masturbated or acted-out in some way, the feeling would go away and you never knew what the real need was and therefore couldn't be responsible to meet that real need. In recovery and to maintain your recovery, you must not only become aware of your feelings and needs, you must take responsibility for them as well. Your wife is not responsible if you feel alone, confused, overwhelmed, or frustrated. You are responsible for your feelings and the needs those feelings create. You need to come up with alternatives to meet your needs in a healthy way.

EXAMPLE:

In addiction:

1. I don't know the feeling > I act out > The feeling goes away

In recovery:

1. I know the feeling > I create need > I am aware and responsible to meet need > My need gets met

Action:

I feel alone > I need to connect with someone > I make phone call > I'm no longer feeling alone

EXERCISE # 55

MY WIFE

Your wife has probably suffered in many ways from your addiction possibly including tolerating your inability to be emotionally intimate, accepting financial losses, humiliation and the list goes on. If your wife is deciding to work this out with you as you recover, you are very fortunate.

"What should I tell my wife?" is one of the first questions I hear from an addict who wants to protect his marriage. The answer is situational. I will offer the following possible options. You may need a therapy session to help you personally in this area.

OPTIONS

1. Tell your wife everything.
2. Tell your wife selective information.
3. Tell vaguely without details "I had an affair."
4. Never tell.

Another issue after you decide to tell or not to tell your spouse is, how much do you include your spouse in your recovery process. In most cases, your spouse will not be a sex addict and will not understand your fantasy, masturbation, pornography or other behavioral struggles. Your spouse is not your sponsor. Your sponsor needs to be someone of the same sex. It is helpful for your spouse to be aware of where you are in your recovery. You may want to agree on some questions your spouse can ask you that you will answer honestly.

Examples of the types of questions you may want to suggest that your spouse may ask about your recovery on a weekly or biweekly agreed upon basis are:

1. Have you crossed your bottom line?
2. Have you masturbated?
3. How often are you going to meetings?
4. Review the five commandments: Prayer, reading, call, meetings, prayer
5. Have you acted-out with another person?

In my experience with other sex addicts, it is a good idea to plan a weekly or biweekly meeting with your wife to discuss these questions. This can prevent your wife from coming up with questions at anytime or during an argument. If your spouse is staying with you during your recovery, it is appropriate and can be therapeutic for you both to keep it in a manageable session. If you have specific questions about these issues, you may want to speak to a therapist.

EXERCISE # 56

STEP THREE

"Made a decision to turn our life and will over to the care of God as we understood Him."

Making a decision of this magnitude can and should take some time in your recovery process. In Step Two, we were spending time with God, discovering His existence and how this relationship is working out. Having a relationship with God is much like those who get married. First we dated our spouse and eventually over time and experiences we decided to marry them and then followed through with this decision. The decision to marry affected every part of our life: socially, financially, sexually and emotionally. In various other areas, marriage redefined our behaviors and us. Turning your life over to the care of God is a similar experience. It is walking down the aisle with God, and a lifelong commitment to stay in a relationship. This relationship grows over time. The depth of our experience and time together will reinforce our conception of God. As a Christian struggling with sex addiction, turning your sexual desires over to God will be essential. To be willing to accept His interpretation of your needs and trust Him to meet them will be very important. A much more thorough discussion of Step Three is available in the *Steps to Freedom* workbook.

Behaviors that support Step Three are:

	BEHAVIOR	**YES**	**NO**
1.	Prayer	_____	_____
2.	Spiritual reading	_____	_____
3.	Asking God to be involved in every area of your life	_____	_____
4.	Behaviorally follow what you know to be God's will, even when you want it another way	_____	_____

EXERCISE # 57

FIVE YEARS FROM NOW: UNRECOVERED

In the more sober moments of your recovery, it is helpful to reinforce how dangerous your addiction can be. Your addiction has a sneaky way of presenting only pretty pictures when it is luring you back into it's unsuspecting web. Sexual addiction will never tell you how bad it can be to be an addict over a period of years. In your recovery, it is helpful to have a clear counter-picture in your mind to fight your addiction. Imagine what it would be like five years from now without recovery and in an active sex addicted lifestyle where you are hurting yourself along with others. Including your feelings in this picture would be a helpful tool against your addiction.

In the lines below, write out what you think your life would be like if you didn't stay in recovery and went back to an active sex addiction lifestyle. The following situations can be included in your picture. 1) People you would be hanging around, 2) People you wouldn't be seeing (wife/children), 3) Where you would be living, 3) The condition of your marriage, 4) Possibly your next spouse and what would this person be like, 5) Your relationship with your children, 6) Your health and risk of disease, 7) Your job and where your career would be going, 8) The amount of time and energy spent on your addiction, 9) How you would feel about yourself, 10) Your secrets, 11) Your spiritual condition and any other situations you can think of to add to your picture.

My life 5 years from now.

_____

_____

_____

_____

_____

_____

Practice imagining the picture with the emotions you have listed above. Your sex addiction has thousands of pictures with emotions to use against you. Having practiced this picture 2 to 3 times a day for 3-5 days can give you a tool to help you get and stay clean.

EXERCISE # 58

<u>PICTURE YOURSELF: UNRECOVERED</u>

In the space provided, draw a picture of yourself in light of five years without recovery.

Describe yourself:

_____

_____

_____

Describe your feelings:

_____

_____

_____

Commit this picture and the feelings to memory. Practice this picture 2 to 3 times daily for 3 to 5 days. This experience can help you counter the "pretty" picture of your addiction.

EXERCISE # 59

<u>FIVE YEARS FROM NOW: RECOVERING</u>

Fighting your sex addiction with pictures is an effective way to help you combat the times your sex addiction wants to creep back in. Many times your sex addiction tries to sneak back in through pictures. Your addiction knows how your brain works, how powerful pictures are, and that vivid, reinforced pictures are quickly accessible to the brain's memory.

With this in mind, some sex addicts can counter-fight the addiction with painful pictures of their addiction and their bleak future with it. Another picture that is helpful to combat our addiction is the picture of the addict having a successful recovery and enjoying himself, his wife, family, career and other relationships and activities.

As someone who has experienced the positive picture of recovery and living a happy, fulfilling and balanced life, I know this picture helps fight off the addiction when it wants to sneak it's ugly head in. In the space provided below, write out what you think your life would be like if you maintain freedom from your sexual addiction with growth in your life of recovery. The following situations could be included in your response.

1. The friends you would have
2. Your career
3. Your marital status
4. Your relationship with your children
5. Your health and risk of sexual diseases
6. How you feel about yourself
7. Secrets you would have
8. Your spiritual lifestyle
9. Recreational interests or hobbies
10. Anything else you see for yourself in a positive recovery future.

My life in recovery 5 years from now:

_____

_____

_____

_____

_____

Take this picture and practice it 2 to 3 times a day for 3 to 5 days along with the feelings that go with it. This picture can be yours. After the hard work that comes with a healthy recovery, there can be fulfillment in every area of your life, spiritual, emotional, health, marriage, friendship, family and financial. My hope is you experience this picture. I have and I know you can too.

My feelings about this picture:

_____

_____

_____

_____

_____

_____

_____

_____

EXERCISE # 60

<u>PICTURE YOURSELF: RECOVERING</u>

In the space below, draw a picture of yourself after five years of successful recovery.

Describe yourself:

_____

_____

_____

_____

Describe your feelings

_____

_____

_____

_____

Commit this picture to memory along with the feelings you have about it. This, among the other pictures you practice 2 to 3 times each day for 3 to 5 days, can be another positively reinforced picture to keep you in recovery.

EXERCISE # 61

MY FAMILY AND ADDICTION

We know as a researched phenomenon, that addictions often run in families. During your recovery process it may be beneficial to do what clinicians call a genogram, which is another name for family tree.

This exercise can be made to be very complicated by listing divorces, etc. but for our purposes, simply draw your family tree with just your family's first names. Take a different colored pen and write next to their name any addiction that you feel this relative may have. A possible list might be alcohol, drugs, sex, gambling, food, television, nicotine, work, shopping and so on. If you are aware of sexual abuse or sexual addiction in your family tree, put an asterisk next to that relative's name as well.

This exercise was developed to help you put your addiction in a family context. This helps you to see that you definitely didn't get where you are all by yourself. In some cases, this can highlight other possible addictions that you may have to look at after a substantial sobriety from sex addiction.

EXERCISE # 62

<u>SEX ADDICTION IN MY FAMILY</u>

The genogram in the last exercise brought to light those in your family with various addictions including sex addiction. In the spaces below, list the family members you feel have sexual addiction issues and why? Secondly, list those who you think were sexually abused in your family tree and why? If you believe no one in your family has had either issue, you may be very fortunate or you just may not have all the information (some families keep better secrets than others.)

<u>NAME/RELATIONSHIP</u>   **<u>WHY</u>**

1. _____   _____

2. _____   _____

3. _____   _____

4. _____   _____

5. _____   _____

6. _____   _____

7. _____   _____

8. _____   _____

9. _____   _____

10. _____   _____

While specifically looking at sexual addiction and abuse, you can sometimes see generationally how this addiction has been carried throughout the family. In my family, sex addiction and sexual abuse are on both sides of my family tree. Those that were in recovery from A.A. in the 1930s when Alcoholics Anonymous just started had this same realization. They knew the addiction was in the family, but the knowledge about the disease wasn't available. The support groups were not there, and there certainly was not a book like the one you are reading that could help them step by step to make recovery their choice. Many in your family history had few choices of recovery or healing from sexual addiction. Write down your thoughts and feelings about possibly being the first in your family to be able to choose this recovery.

EXERCISE # 63

MY SEXUAL HISTORY

A sexual history is something that many sex addicts have stored in their minds. Faces, pictures and events periodically may come into your mind. These pictures sometimes stir up feelings of all different kinds. You may be less than proud of your sexual history but regardless of where you are in your recovery, your sexual history can be a tool to help you see and discover things about yourself and your addiction.

To write a sexual history, get a pen and paper and simply go through your life in increments of 5 years (1-5, 6-10, 11-15, 16-20...). Write down all your sexual experiences. This would include exposure to pornography at various ages, masturbation patterns, and your first sexual experience. This history when done thoroughly will help you when you do your Fourth Step. The temptation will be to avoid complete honesty.

A complete history will have several benefits such as:

1.   It is finally all out.

2.   Great progress toward Fourth Step.

3.   You will be able to do the Sex Cycles Exercise.

EXERCISE # 64

<u>SEX CYCLES AND STRATEGIES</u>

In the previous exercise, you took great courage to write your sexual history down. This is important and can help you identify patterns from your sexual experiences.

Some addicts review their sexual histories and find a series of re-victimizations, or that their first sexual experience was abusive and that they were used as someone's object. Others find cycles of intensity under stress, or right after a major abandonment. You may also find out something about those you chose to be sexual with, such as they were emotionally unavailable or that they were unfaithful. Other sexual experiences might be victimizing others, the continual reliance on masturbation and/or pornography at the expense of relationships. A pattern of being unfulfilled sexually and seeking the magic fix can also emerge. Stress and financial pressure for some are related to sexual cycles. Others can see when they have extra money that they exhibit a pattern of acting-out. Being out of town is a pattern some discover. For some addicts a definite binge-purge pattern emerges where they are "good" for so long and then they act out excessively and binge. There is a myriad of possible sexual cycles. In the below space, briefly write out the cycles you recognize in your sexual history.

_____

_____

_____

Now that you have identified some cycles as they relate to your sexual history, you may for the first time realize the reality of certain cycles or patterns in your acting-out. To make the most of these realizations, it will help if you make a plan or strategy to "short circuit" the patterns that are already in place. For example, if you are out of town, plan to attend a 12-step meeting in that town, cancel movies in your room, take recovery-reading materials and make at least one or two check-in calls a day to your home group members. If you are a binge and purge type, plan to attend more meetings and read and pray more when you sense a binge coming on. Doubling up on calls during this time may be helpful strategies to avoid the binge cycle. In the below section, write your recovery strategies.

_____

_____

_____

EXERCISE # 65

TYPES OF SEX

The types of sex listed below are excerpts taken from the book *Women Who Love Sex Addicts*. This approach can help you to see the type of sex you have had with your wife. The sex addict is often amazed that after 5-10 or more years of objectifying or maybe masturbating sex, that his spouse isn't interested that much in sex. Many sex addicts and their wives have rarely even had *relational* sex in their entire marriage.

The awareness of the types of sex can help you in your recovery to aim for *relational* sex in your recovery. It also will help you to be empathetic to the type of sex you have conditioned yourself and your wife to have over the years of your relationship. In recovery, you can have a growing sexual relationship that is not only relational but also nurturing and fulfilling as well.

Relational Sex: Both enjoy each other as a person, and are able to communicate sexual needs to one another. One or both may or may not have an orgasm, but both have a sense of nurturing each other. Sex is not the focus or the priority in this relationship.

Physical Sex: This is where one or both enjoy primarily the physical act, but still the relationship is not threatened. This type of sex may happen at one time or another to all couples. There may not be much feeling but shame is not a factor.

Objectifying Sex: This type of sex may or may not be pleasurable for the wife. The addict is fantasizing about other sexual acts with his wife. One person's orgasm is the focus of this type of sexual act. The wife may or may not feel important to the orgasmic partner.

Masturbating Sex: The addict is fantasizing about the either the other person, pornographic movies, books, or someone else, while having sex with his wife. The primary focus is the person having the orgasm, not his wife. The wife may feel used, absent, or resentful of this sexual encounter.

Violating Sex: This is where the addict demands certain behaviors from his wife while she does not feel comfortable performing them. Although the wife complies, she hopes the addict will stop requesting this particular sexual act. The wife feels violated as a person, and may have anger or resentment toward him for insisting on this particular sexual activity.

Traumatizing Sex: The wife is forced physically or with the threat of a weapon or physical pain, to perform a sexual act with the addict. This constitutes rape, and the woman may feel incredible fear of the perpetrator, as well as feelings of victimization and trauma.

EXERCISE # 66

SEXUAL SYSTEMS

As couples evolve together, they create systems for various aspects of their relationship such as who manages the money, who takes the children to school, and who takes out the garbage. Some couples create shared systems, or systems may evolve in which one person has total responsibility for one specific area.

It is not uncommon for the sex addict, who may initiate sex more frequently than his wife to end up being totally responsible for the sexual relationship. This leads to discussions such as "you never initiate sex." Her response to this may be "you never give me time to." This also leads to the fact that if the addict does all the initiating, he is going to receive 100% of the rejections to be sexual no matter how few times this may actually be.

Systems as they evolve with couples happen slowly and over time. The system around sex is rarely discussed and hence usually does not change. Some of the different sex systems that can be created are listed below.

1. Solo System - Only one person initiates sex, takes all the risk and receives the refusals. This system can lead to only one person's sexual needs being held as being important.
2. Scheduled System - The couple decides the frequency of sex they want, whether it is once or several times a week, and a particular partner initiates sex on certain nights.
3. Shared System - Both partners are equally responsible for the sexual initiating. The couple decides how to break this up by days, weeks or months.
4. Rotating System - In this system, both partners are responsible to initiate. The couple chooses the frequency of sexual encounters desired in a week or month and then rotates who is responsible to initiate. For example: James and Robin choose to have sex twice a week. They decide to rotate who initiates on a 3-day schedule. When it is James's turn to initiate, he has three days to manage a convenient time for both of them. When he has initiated, the next day begins Robin's turn to initiate. Neither partner has to wait till the last day to initiate. Couples like this system because they feel more opportunities to be spontaneous within the system.

In the above-mentioned systems, it is not uncommon during the development for one or both partners to be aggressive or passive/aggressive in an attempt to resist the change. Some addicts don't like giving up total control of their sex lives and some wives don't want any sexual responsibility. If this occurs, a system of consequences can be set up for the system you both select. This can be a very sensitive topic. You may need some professional guidance in this area to come to an agreed upon system and to create consequences or a sense of guidance as you go through this process.

EXERCISE # 67

SEXUAL ASSERTIVENESS

To talk to a sex addict about sexual assertiveness may seem to be an oxymoron. In the sex addict's addiction lifestyle, he may have been sexually aggressive, passive or manipulative, but rarely assertive.

Being sexually aggressive, demanding or sometimes forceful on your wife is not healthy and can leave life-long scars on her. The sexually passive sex addict usually takes care of his sexual needs by being sexual with himself or being involved in sexual activity outside the relationship. While this is going on, the sex addict may avoid his wife's sexual needs. Depriving your wife of her sexual needs also is unhealthy. Usually in this passive system, the wife has to initiate the sexual encounter. This could also mean the sex addict is also sexually anorexic.

The sexual manipulativeness of the sex addict is by far the most prevalent sexual arrangement I see with couples. In this arrangement, hints, winks, massages, touches or a sexual comment is supposed to be interpreted by her as "I would like to have sex with you." Since these hints or comments are not direct, they can be misunderstood and hence you may go away mad because you thought your wife should be able to read your mind by your manipulations toward wanting to have sex. This system leaves a lot to interpret and can lead to many "you knew what I meant" arguments about sex.

Sexual <u>assertiveness</u> includes two aspects. The first aspect is asking **directly** to be sexual with your wife. The second aspect is having respect for your wife and realizing that just because you asked for sex doesn't mean you are entitled to what you asked for.

To practice sexual assertiveness, ask your wife to sit in a chair in front of you and simply practice several times asking her directly to be sexual. Remember this is just a practice. Do not actually initiate sex at this time otherwise it may feel as if you are being manipulative with her. In this exercise, it is not necessary for your wife to have any response. After you have asked her several times, switch and allow her to ask you the same question. Remember this is a practice exercise. Responding in an inappropriate manner may block the progress this exercise can give you. This exercise can be practiced once or twice a day until both of you feel comfortable asking the other to be sexual. Statements that have worked for other couples are as follows.

- ❑ I would like to be sexual with you, would that be convenient for you?
- ❑ I am feeling sexual and would like to be sexual with you. Can we do this?
- ❑ Can we be sexual together?
- ❑ Is being sexual with you an option today or tonight?

NOTE: Do not practice this exercise in the bedroom or at a time you would normally have sex.

EXERCISE # 68

REJECTION DESENSITIZATION
(Learning to Say "No")

Saying "no" to the sex addict regarding sexual relations can create a big problem for him. This problem has a long history and an explainable origin. In most of the sex addicts fantasy and masturbation habits possibly since early adolescence, he rarely heard the word "no." This distorted reality that every time he wants to ejaculate he had an willing partner (his fantasy), created a distorted conditioning. In reality, a healthy wife may not desire sex every single time he wants it. After clocking in hundreds of hours confirming a fantasy with an ejaculation, the sex addict really believes that the fantasy is reality.

This is what causes the sex addict to blow up and get mad and sometimes find ways to "get even" when his wife says "no, not tonight." Some sex addicts go into total rages when rejected sexually. The sex addict's conditioning is the problem, not his wife.

When your wife says "no, not tonight," she is not saying "I hate you." This is the way some sex addicts interpret what she is saying and it is not reality. So as an addict, you may need to do some desensitization to realize that your wife is not rejecting you as a person (core belief of a sex addict is that you are your sex), but rather she just is not wanting to participate with you sexually at this particular time. She knows that there are going to be other times to be sexual together.

The following exercise is a way to help you accept the variety of responses you may get from your wife without blowing up after a rejection. It also helps the wife to practice asking for sexual intimacy rather than the addict doing 100% of the asking. Do this exercise at a time you would not normally have sex and preferably not in the bedroom. You and your wife sit face to face, maintaining eye contact. Ask your wife if you can be sexual with her (see assertiveness exercise). She is to have three responses, which are noted below.

YOU		WIFE'S RESPONSE
Would you like to be sexual?	1.	Yes, I would like to have sex with you.
Would you like to be sexual?	2.	I would like to be sexual at a later time.
Would you like to be sexual?	3.	No, I do not want to be sexual at this time.

Practice this several times in one setting asking a total of nine times. Then switch and have your wife ask and you give the responses above. This exercise will probably have to be done 10 to 14 times to get some level of desensitization.

List below the dates you have practiced this exercise:

_____ _____ _____ _____ _____ _____ _____ _____

_____ _____ _____ _____ _____ _____ _____ _____

91

EXERCISE # 69

SEX TALK

During sexual encounters, it is not uncommon for sex addicts to disconnect and go into various levels of fantasy states. As you recover and want a healthier and more satisfying sex life, it is important that you nurture and communicate relationally with your wife during your sexual act. The response I so often get from sex addicts is "what do I say while being sexual?" Below is a list of relational statements that may help you through this dilemma.

❑ I love you.

❑ I really have more love for you now than ever.

❑ Thank you for sharing yourself with me.

❑ You're a terrific lover.

❑ I enjoy being with you.

❑ I feel close to you.

❑ I desire you.

❑ I'm glad I'm with you.

❑ I'm proud of you.

❑ I love looking at you.

❑ You are such a comfort to me.

❑ I like growing with you.

❑ I love my life with you.

❑ I thank God you're my wife.

❑ Thank you for loving me.

❑ You are a neat person.

❑ I like you.

❑ I'm glad I married you.

❑ You're beautiful.

❑ I love your eyes.

EXERCISE # 70

SEX: SPIRIT, SOUL, AND BODY

Sex is tridimensional. It is one of the few activities that can touch all three parts of your being: spirit, soul, and body. As a sex addict, you may have been emotionally and spiritually underdeveloped due to your addiction. Most sex addicts have only experienced sex in one dimension and that is physically, which may explain the need for more sex almost immediately after having sex. The sex addict desires three-dimensional sex but is not currently available for this experience.

Most sex addicts feel they may have perfected the biological aspect of sex. This one-dimensional aspect of sex is what I call "water gun" sex. The development of the other two areas of our being has to occur for us to reach three-dimensional sex. If you are early in your recovery, you may not have any experiential reference point for what I am talking about. After several months into your recovery, you may smile and say "Oh, that's what he was talking about." After a longer period of sobriety and much hard work in emotional and spiritual development many sex addicts will finally have three-dimensional sex.

Tips to working through this three-dimensional sexual process are:

1. Feelings work.
2. Pray alone.
3. Pray with your wife.
4. Share your feelings with your wife.
5. Act in a responsible way toward your wife (do what you say)
6. Practice sexual assertiveness and sex tips in this book.

93

EXERCISE # 71

<u>SEX TIPS</u>

During your growing transformation from objectifying sex to relational sex, there are some tips that may help the process get easier. These tips are for you to practice during your sexual encounters to make it more fulfilling for both you and your wife.

Tip #1: <u>Keep Your Eyes Open</u> - Keeping your eyes open during intercourse makes disconnecting and fantasizing for either spouse more difficult. Disconnecting is the first step to fantasy. Being present emotionally during sex may be uncomfortable at first but will become easier as you both practice.

Tip #2: <u>Keep the Lights On</u> - Having some light on during the sexual encounter is helpful in two ways. First, if it was dark, you couldn't tell, nor would it matter, if your eyes were open since you couldn't see anyway. Secondly, you can keep eye contact with your wife which will again keep you from disconnecting and going into fantasy.

Tip #3: <u>Relational Conversation</u> - Having relational conversation (i.e., I love you. You are beautiful.) will also keep you focussed on the present sexual encounter. Stay away from inappropriate talk, although familiar to many sex addicts, it may reinforce your addictive, objectifying sex as opposed to reinforcing relational sex with your wife.

EXERCISE # 72

MY SEX PLAN

In the space below, write out what you believe is your sexual plan. This will help you to be very clear as to what are the current parameters of your sexuality for you and your wife.

Behaviors my wife and I agree upon are:

_____

_____

_____

The frequency my wife and I agree to are:

_____

Our agreed upon method of asking for sex is:

_____

The responsibility for asking for sex is:

_____

Parameters for where we will have sex are:

_____

_____

_____

EXERCISE # 73

PROFESSIONAL COUNSELING

There are several different types of counselors available. Few professionals in the mental health field are aware of or familiar with sexual addiction treatment at this time. Questions to ask a therapist you would consider for counseling are at the end of this exercise. You may want to consider our counseling services mentioned in the back of this book. For those not living within the local area, our services include telephone counseling as well or see the Appendix for video therapy information.

Along the path of recovery it may be important or necessary for you to get professional help. This can be a scary enough reality for you. To find someone who is qualified in the area of sexual addiction is essential if the counseling is going to be beneficial for your recovery. The stories of what untrained counselors, regardless if they were psychiatrists or psychologists or master's level counselors, have told people trying to recover from sex addiction is astounding.

This is why we have prepared some questions to ask your therapist or doctor before you agree to see them. First, it is important to note that psychiatrists are medical doctors whose primary solution for their client is medicine. Psychologists, social workers and master's level counselors are more counseling oriented in their solutions for their clients. The questions you may want to ask are:

1. How much experience do you have working with sexual addiction?
2. How much of your practice is related to sexual addiction?
3. Do you have specialized training/certification/licensure in addictions?
4. Are you a recovering person who has worked the 12 Steps personally?
5. What books have you read related to sex addiction?
6. Do you have specific training dealing with sexual abuse issues?

These six questions can be a starter for you to assess the professional you desire to hire to help you recover from your sexual addiction. It is possible, however, in your geographical area to not have a therapist who specializes in sexual addiction.

EXERCISE # 74

<u>READ A BOOK ON CO-SEX ADDICTION</u>

If you are a sex addict, why should you read a book on co-addiction? Many sex addicts have selected co-addicts as spouses. The co-addiction system works out well when married to a sex addict. There is a need for change for both spouses in the marital system during your recovery process.

Co-addicts, in general, have little difficulty in buying books on sex addiction and reading them. It can even be the case that in a short period of time, she may know more about your addiction than her own. The co-addict's book will help you understand the co-addict and the struggles she may have.

The anger she may have toward you is normal. The grief she goes through is also normal. The recovery she will have to go through is a process. The more informed you are about her, the better you will understand that both of you need to recover so you can both experience a healthy marriage in recovery as opposed to a marriage in addiction. Co-addiction books you may want to pick from are available through Heart to Heart Counseling Center. An order form is available in the back of this book. Books that would be especially helpful are:

Women Who Love Sex Addicts	By Weiss	$14.95
Affair of the Mind	By Hall	$14.95
Partner's Recovery Guide	By Weiss	$39.95
Beyond Love (wkbk)	By Weiss	$14.95

EXERCISE # 75

<u>STEP FOUR</u>

"Made a searching and fearless inventory of ourselves."

Making a personal inventory is helpful in many ways. Firstly, an inventory tells you what has happened and when it happened, both good and harmful. Secondly, this inventory will give you insight into patterns or cycles of unhealthy behavior. Without this "spreadsheet" you would not be able to see clearly. There are several ways to complete a Fourth step, but all include in one way or another writing it down somewhere.

Let's define a few terms first, such as the word "good" which indicates positive things that happened. "Bad" will mean things that you did that you knew were wrong and did them despite this knowledge. A lot of addiction history will fall into this category. "Ugly" will be things that happened to you that you weren't responsible for such as car accidents, surgeries, parent's divorce, abuse or neglect. With these terms in mind, take a piece of paper and draw your columns and a place for the span of years as seen below and fill in "the rest of the story." Below are some examples.

<u>YEARS</u>	<u>GOOD</u>	<u>BAD</u>	<u>UGLY</u>
1-5			
6-10	won spelling bee		placed in foster home
11-15		stole porn	
16-20...			

Behaviors that support a Step Four are as follows.

<u>BEHAVIOR</u>		<u>YES</u>	<u>NO</u>
1.	Consistent time spent writing your story	_____	_____
2.	Complete honesty on your story	_____	_____
3.	Checking in if memories affect sobriety	_____	_____

EXERCISE # 76

STEP FIVE

"Admitted to God, ourselves, and to another human being the exact nature of our wrongs."

In Step Four, you provided yourself with all the information you need to do your Step Five. Step Four is "your" story. It is a story that has shadows much like others who are recovering from sexual addiction. This story needs to be admitted to yourself which usually happens during the writing, reading, or sharing of your Fourth Step.

"Admitting to God," for some has been an event all by itself. God already knows, but something can happen when you tell Him where you have been. Some addicts visually put God in an empty chair and read their story to Him. This may be a helpful exercise to do in your Fifth Step process.

Having "another human being" involved is by far the toughest part. To allow someone else into your closet of secrets is difficult but entirely necessary for your fullest recovery from sexual addiction. Pick a person in the recovery program, a support person of the same sex (not your spouse), or a pastor or therapist to share your story with.

The Fifth Step is a must in your recovery from sexual addiction. While finishing your Fifth Step, you will feel less guilt and shame and experience acceptance even though you once believed that "if someone really knew me, they wouldn't love me." This isn't true and in your Fifth Step, you will get to experience being human, flaws and all.

Behaviors that support a Fifth Step are as follows.

BEHAVIORS	**YES**	**NO**
1. A written down Fourth Step	_____	_____
2. A time of reflecting with yourself "admitting to yourself"	_____	_____
3. A time you and God go through "admitting to yourself"	_____	_____
4. Picking someone to share your Fifth Step with	_____	_____
5. Making an appointment to share "your story"	_____	_____
6. Sharing your Story	_____	_____

The day I completed my Fifth Step was _____.

EXERCISE # 77

<u>SPONSORING OTHERS</u>

Sponsoring, or discipling others can be a vital part of your personal recovery from sexual addiction. I can't tell you how many times God has spoken through me to someone in recovery needing help. In the scripture, Jesus stated that in a situation where people are being restored, there He is. I am glad that I have been called to this ministry. Helping another struggling sex addict will strengthen your faith and remind you of the precious gift you have been given in your recovery.

My experience is that when a Christian gets his sexual addiction into submission, he is truly free and has the ability, by example, to free others. My hope is that as you heal, pass the healing along to others.

EXERCISE # 78

HIV TEST

The reality of AIDS is everywhere. As an addict, you definitely need to be aware of your possible risk. If your sexual behaviors have included other people than your wife, you definitely need an AIDS test. This is not just for your piece of mind, but so that you know you are not continually exposing your wife to a possible life threatening disease. This test can be done anonymously in most of the larger cities in our country. The results take anywhere from a couple days to a couple weeks.

The exercise of getting an AIDS test has brought some soberness to many addicts and their wives if they get tested as well. There is nothing quite like a community clinic to bring home how your life has become out of control and how very much you have to lose if you continue in your addiction.

Going to an AIDS clinic is like a speeding addict going to court for a speeding ticket without a lawyer. There is the reality that what the addict has been doing is harmful and there is the fact that he may actually get consequences for his behavior. Unlike the speeding addict, our consequence may be our own health and life and that of our spouse's as well.

If you need added support to go through this exercise, recruit a recovering person to go to the clinic with you both times. This exercise can also give tremendous relief when the results are negative.

EXERCISE # 79

GROWING UP

Growing Up Sexually

You have learned a lot of things growing up in your family. Some of the things you learned are helpful and some are not so helpful. This exercise is going to focus on your family's sexual education. As a child or adolescent, you were taught not only by what your parents said and did but also the attitudes and unwritten rules your parents believed in.

What did you learn about sex from Mom and Dad?

Mom: _____

_____

_____

Dad: _____

_____

_____

From the above information, what beliefs or behaviors you have duplicated in your life. List them below:

_____

_____

_____

What were the long-term results of the sexual beliefs or behaviors that you saw in your parent's life or relationship?

_____

_____

_____

What specific plans can you make to not duplicate these same results in your life and relationships?

_____

_____

_____

How to Treat Members of the Opposite Sex

How you treat yourself and others is usually to some degree what you have seen or experienced in your family of origin. A client recently discovered after 40 years that he created the exact non-intimate relationship that his parents had. His personal way of relating had a great deal to do with this.

Patterns of relating to your wife are taught by your perceptions of your parent's relationship. This can definitely be the case in what you learned about treating your wife. In the spaces below, write what you learned about treating the opposite sex, both beliefs and behaviors from:

Dad: _____

_____

Mom: _____

_____

From the above lists, are there any beliefs or behaviors you have duplicated in your life? If so list them below.

_____

_____

What were the long-term results of these beliefs or behaviors about treating others?

_____

_____

What specific plan can you make not to duplicate these results in your life and relationships?

_____

_____

Growing Up With Anger

Anger is one thing very few people talk about. As a recovering sex addict, you will need to discuss and deal with anger from several perspectives. In this section, you will be focusing on what you learned about anger from your parents. In some families, you can only discuss feelings after you get mad. In other words, it is okay to hit or be verbally abusive if you are mad. Many rules about anger are learned in the home such as don't get mad, ever. Instead, eat or drink alcohol to cope with your anger, run away, withdraw or emotionally punish others with your anger. In the space below, list what you learned about anger, regarding beliefs and behaviors from your Mom and Dad.

Mom: _____

_____

Dad: _____

_____

From the above list, are there any beliefs or behaviors you have duplicated in your life? If so list them:

_____

_____

What were the long-term results of these beliefs or behaviors about anger that you saw in your parent's life-style or relationship in the future?

_____

_____

What specific plan can you make not to duplicate these results in your lifestyle and relationship?

_____

_____

EXERCISE # 80

MY RELATIONSHIP WITH DAD

In the space provided, describe your relationship with your Dad as you remember it <u>as a child</u>.

_____

_____

_____

_____

In the space provided, write down what your relationship with your Dad was as you remember it <u>as a teenager</u>.

_____

_____

_____

In the space provided, describe your relationship with your Dad <u>as an adult</u>.

_____

_____

_____

_____

I feel happy about my relationship with Dad because _____

_____

_____

I feel sad about my relationship with Dad because _____

_____

_____

I feel mad about my relationship with Dad because _____

_____

_____

My hope for my relationship with Dad is _____

_____

_____

_____

In the space below, write a letter to your dad. This letter is for therapeutic purposes only. It is not to be sent to him or seen by him unless you discuss it with your sponsor or therapist. You can express any feelings or situations in your letter, and it may be longer than the space provided.

_____

_____

_____

_____

_____

_____

At different times in your recovery, you will need to confront specific issues. The work you have done in the last few pages may have been difficult and emotional. Your courage to be honest will be a great asset in your recovery.

To confront some of these family of origin issues, it is not necessary that you actually go see your parents and drag up all the stuff that you have been processing and try to dump it on them in a one-time conversation. Dumping on them doesn't have to occur for you to get better or even to confront the past issues. What you are about to do may be also very difficult and emotional. If you feel you may need support by a recovering person or therapist, please get it.

Take the "Dear Dad" letter that you wrote and sit in a chair with another chair facing you. When you are ready, take your letter to Dad, read it as if he were right there in the chair across from you. You may or may not experience a wide variety of feelings during this exercise.

This empty chair exercise can further your sense of expression toward your Dad as well as give you a sense of confronting past feelings or issues. Having these issues addressed can leave you less vulnerable in your sex addiction recovery.

EXERCISE # 81

MY RELATIONSHIP WITH MOM

In the space provided, describe your relationship with your Mom as you remember it <u>as a child.</u>

_____

_____

_____

In the space below, write down what your relationship with your Mom was like <u>as a teenager.</u>

_____

_____

_____

In the space below, describe your relationship with your Mom <u>as an adult.</u>

_____

_____

_____

I feel happy about my relationship with Mom because_____

_____

_____

I feel sad about my relationship with Mom because_____

_____

_____

I feel mad about my relationship with Mom because_____

_____

My hopes for my relationship with Mom are_____

_____

_____

    In the space below, write a letter to your mother. This letter is for therapeutic purposes only and is not to be sent to her or seen by her unless you run it by a therapist or your sponsor. You can express any feelings or situations in your letter, and it can be much longer than the space provided.

_____

_____

_____

_____

_____

    This exercise is similar to the empty chair exercise you did for Dad. Take your "Dear Mom" letter and sit in a chair with another chair facing you while imagining that she is sitting in the chair. When you are ready, take your letter to Mom and read it as if she were sitting across from you. You may or may not experience a wide variety of feelings during this exercise.

    This empty chair can further your sense of expression toward Mom as well as give you a sense of confronting past feelings or issues. Having these issues addressed can leave you less vulnerable in your recovery.

EXERCISE # 82

<u>MY RELATIONSHIP WITH GOD</u>

Now here is someone you may or may not have met growing up. In your family, your parents may have made God important in a healthy way, a religiously unhealthy way, occasionally important (i.e., holidays and emergencies) or not important at all. No matter what your family did or did not do to introduce you to God, many have their own unique development with God.

In this exercise, you will want to look at what you learned about God from your parents. In the space below, describe what you believe to be your parent's belief and behaviors about God.

Mom's belief and behaviors about God: _____

_____

_____

Dad's belief and behaviors about God: _____

_____

_____

From the above information, are there any beliefs or behaviors that you have duplicated in your life? If so, what are they?

_____

_____

_____

What were the long-term effects of these beliefs or behaviors (good or bad) that you saw in your parent's life or relationship?

_____

_____

_____

What specific plan can you make to avoid these negative results in your life and relationship?

_____

_____

In the space below, describe your relationship with God <u>as a child:</u>

_____

_____

In the space below, describe your relationship with God <u>as a teenager:</u>

_____

_____

In the space below, describe your relationship with God <u>as an adult:</u>

_____

_____

Describe your relationship with God as an adult prior to your recovery from sexual addiction.

_____

_____

In the space provided below, describe your relationship with God as a recovering person.

_____

_____

_____

I'm glad about my relationship with God because: _____

_____

_____

I'm sad about my relationship with God because: _____

_____

_____

I'm mad about my relationship with God because: _____

_____

_____

My wishes about my relationship with God are: _____

_____

_____

_____

In the space below, write a letter to God.

_____

_____

_____

_____

_____

Since we all come from a variety of backgrounds, God may be different for all of us. This exercise may not be necessary for all sex addicts, but most of you will be helped by "a talk with God". In the past pages dealing with family of origin issues, you imagined sitting both Mom and Dad in a chair in front of you and confronted the issues you felt you had with your parents.

In this exercise, you can do the same confronting of your issues with God. God can be a big relationship in your past as well as in your recovery. Being yourself before God is very important in order to move further in your spirituality and relationship with God.

In light of this, take your "Dear God" letter and place yourself in a chair along with a chair in front of you. Imagine God sitting in the chair in front of you. Read your letter to God and say anything else you feel impressed to say to Him. This exercise for some may be difficult and may make you feel a wide variety of emotions. If you feel you need the support of a recovering person or a therapist please do this for your personal well being.

EXERCISE # 83

ABUSES AND NEGLECTS

During your Fourth Step, you made a column titled "ugly." In this section of your Fourth Step, you listed events that happened to you that were not your fault although they still impacted your life. It is now time to look at these events and begin healing from them as a part of your sexual addiction recovery.

Many sex addicts have experienced various forms of abuse. Some **emotional abuse** instances could consist of being shamed, degraded, humiliated or yelled at regularly. **Emotional neglect** could involve not being talked to, nurtured, nor having someone care as to how you feel. They may not inquire about your feelings. **Physical abuse** would include hitting or watching others being hit. **Physical neglect** would include being improperly clothed or not having adequate food or shelter. **Spiritual abuse** is sometimes being emotionally or physically abused while your parents justify this by their religious beliefs. Some **sexual abuse** instances would include exposure to pornography, verbal sexual innuendoes, sexual touches and other behaviors. **Sexual neglect** is not informing you about your body changes and about sex.

In the space provided below, check the areas of abuse and or neglects you feel you have experienced:

ABUSES		NEGLECTS	
Emotional	_____	Emotional	_____
Physical	_____	Physical	_____
Spiritual	_____	Spiritual	_____
Sexual	_____	Sexual	_____

EXERCISE # 84

<u>MY PERPETRATORS</u>

In the previous exercise, you took a look at the abuses and neglects you May have experienced. In this exercise, you are going to look at the people who were responsible for these abuses and neglects.

I know at this point, you may be going into very painful territory. So painful that many of these issues may be the very pains you were medicating by acting out sexually. It is very important to your healing process that you look at these abuses and neglects that you suffered.

In many of the incidences that you have experienced, you may have known the perpetrator's name. For some, these events happened in your own home by parents, stepparents, siblings or extended family. In other cases, there may be a casual relationship that proceeded the abuse (i.e. a schoolteacher, another child at school, or neighbor). For some, the person may be a stranger and you may not know the perpetrator's name. Maybe it only happened once and you never saw them again.

Whatever their name or relationship was, these events have been indelibly written into your life. Now it is time to write down your perpetrator's name (if known), relationship (if any), and the type of abuse that occurred and an approximate age that the abuse/neglect happened.

NAME / RELATIONSHIP   ABUSE / NEGLECT   AGE

_____

_____

_____

_____

_____

_____

_____

EXERCISE # 85

WHAT YOU DID TO ME

What you may have experienced from your perpetrator(s) has most likely left you with a lot pain for probably many years. This pain is often free-floating inside of you. You may rarely or never talk about what exactly happened and so it may remain like an emotional blob of gel that you don't seem to have crystallized inside.

In your recovery, it will be important to feel this pain you have been medicating all these years and to crystallize it as much as possible. It will be very helpful in your recovery for you to identify what exactly happened and later to process your feelings about these events.

In this exercise, you will do exactly that. Crystallize the memory. On the previous page you wrote down your perpetrators and their general offenses. It is now time to get specific. On a separate paper list the perpetrator at the top of the page and write down in as much detail as you possibly can exactly what your perpetrator did.

If you have experienced sexual, physical or other abuses, this will be painful. If you need the support of others, please call and invite others into this healing process with you. If you feel you need professional help at this point, consider a therapist who specializes in this area of recovery.

EXERCISE # 86

RANKING MY PERPETRATOR (S)

Ranking your perpetrator may seem like an odd thing to do, after all, any abuse no matter what kind should never be experienced by anybody. I know this as well as anyone. And in ranking, you are not trying to minimize in any way the pain each perpetrator has inflicted on your life.

I compare the exercise process before you to the work of a battle surgeon. Every wound that a soldier has is painful and yet some wounds will require different levels of procedures and some wounds may demand more attention than others. While completing the letter and anger work to be done ahead, proceed by ranking the perpetrators in your perception as to which has caused more damage and pain so we can outline a plan for surgery.

In this exercise, you will need to categorize from the perpetrator ranked least abusive and work up to the major traumas that will require harder work from you in the exercises ahead of you. By working in a ranked order starting with the least traumatic, you will be stronger and know the process and what to expect a lot better as you move into the higher ranked trauma events.

On the previous page where you listed your perpetrators, the abuse/neglect and their age, write next to their name a rank, starting with the #1 as the least offending, moving up to the most severe as the highest ranked abuse.

EXERCISE # 87

<u>LETTER(S) TO MY PERPETRATOR(S)</u>

This exercise takes you a step further into healing from your abuses and/or neglects that you may have experienced. Much like you have already done in creating letters to help you resolve some of the family of origin issues, you now must write a letter to help heal these areas of abuse and neglect.

This letter to each of your perpetrators is for therapeutic purposes, not to be sent to the perpetrator(s). These letters are for your recovery, not theirs. It is important for you to confront the issue but not necessarily the person, especially at this time of recovery. You may have a wide range of feelings as you do this exercise. You may want to solicit the help of a support person and stay in closer touch with your group during this time.

In this exercise, imagine having your perpetrator in a room, strapped to a chair. Imagine that they couldn't say anything to you and you could say anything and everything you wanted to them. This letter can be full of hate, anger, disgust and many include other powerful emotions. You can use any language necessary to express yourself. These events should have never happened, so your feelings are totally appropriate.

These letters can be as long as you need in order to fully express yourself. These letters can bring up past feelings and memories. Give yourself permission to feel them and take as much time as you need. You are worth the time and energy you will need to take on your letters.

Now write down the name of the perpetrator that you ranked "least" on the previous page, and begin to write your letter. After you write your letter, you may want to do an empty chair exercise and read your letter to the perpetrator. If you feel you need a support person present while doing this exercise, please do this for yourself.

If after reading the letter, you feel a sense of resolve, that's great. If you feel there is more work to do, then you may want to consider further assistance from a therapist or support person. There is a specific therapeutic experiential exercise you can do to relieve trauma issues. This exercise needs to be worked through with a therapist. I have seen many relieved from past physical and sexual trauma issues through this technique offered in our counseling center. Sex addicts do well to resolve their trauma issues especially for those where it is the fuel that feeds their addiction.

EXERCISE # 88

STEP SIX

"Were entirely ready to have God remove all these defects of character."

Defects of character may be more obvious to you now that you have written and acknowledged your story to God, yourself and another human being. In Step Six, you can begin to see some of your limitations or things that are less than positive about yourself. Before you can become "entirely ready," it has been helpful for many sex addicts to take some reflective time and list your defects of character. Writing down your defects (i.e., impatient, manipulative, selfish) helps you to know what it is that you are getting ready to have God remove.

The simplest way to do this is to list in the left-hand column your <u>character defects</u>. Next to the character defect, write the <u>percentage that you are willing to have God remove this defect,</u> (EXAMPLE: Selfishness - 75%). Review your list regularly until there is a 100% next to each defect. During the starting of this list and it's completion you may want to pray over those areas that are less than 100% ready.

Behaviors supporting a Step Six are as follows.

BEHAVIORS	**YES**	**NO**
1. A list of "defects of character"	_____	_____
2. A regular review until 100% "entirely ready"	_____	_____
3. Prayer during the process of becoming "entirely ready"	_____	_____
4. Discussions about defects taking longer to be "entirely ready"	_____	_____

Date I became entirely ready to have God remove my defects of character _____.

119

EXERCISE # 89

STEP SEVEN

"Humbly asked Him to remove our shortcomings."

You may be very familiar with your shortcomings. Being too familiar with your short-comings can sometimes make it difficult to get into a humble place and ask God to remove them. In my life, my shortcomings hurt those I loved very much and looking back, these same shortcomings hurt me, too. Shortcomings often need a real miracle to be removed.

I liken this process to that of your child, parent, or spouse who might suddenly be diagnosed with a life threatening disease and all the doctor had to say is "if you pray, now is a good time to do so." Many sex addicts, regardless of their life history or circumstances, would muster up a "humble asking" position before God. If someone was watching you, they might call it begging, pleading for God to be merciful "just this once." This is the place to be while completing your Seventh Step.

Asking God to remove your shortcomings is very hard spiritual work. While working on Step Seven, you may want to seriously consider completing just one or two defects a day. More than this may be too draining or may minimize this defect. Some have found it helpful to write down a paragraph or two about how a defect of character has hurt them as well as others to assist in humbly asking God to remove them.

Behaviors that support a Step Seven are as follows.

BEHAVIORS	**YES**	**NO**
1. List of defects	_____	_____
2. Paragraph of how defects affect you and those that you love.	_____	_____
3. A reflective time	_____	_____
4. A prayer time for each defect	_____	_____

Date I completed praying over each defect _____.

EXERCISE # 90

<u>THE VICTIMS</u>

In any addiction, there are going to be victims. Each addict has led a secret life. In the secret life you lived in, there may be people that you have victimized. You may have victimized sexual partners, your wife or even your children or other people's children.

These victimizations play a heavy role in guilt and shame. Every day you may live with the faces of innocent people you victimized. In your recovery, there comes a place to deal specifically with the sexual or nonsexual pain you may have caused.

Write down the first names of those you victimized. Place the names and the approximate age you violated them. Keep the work you are doing in a safe place. The courage you take to face the issues of your sexual inappropriate behavior and victimizations will help you maintain the precious sobriety you have worked so hard for. The past is the past, but you can not be sober and minimize the pain you may have caused others.

EXERCISE # 91

<u>HOW I HURT THEM</u>

Take the paper you used from the previous exercise and write down your violation to them. Take as much time as you need to fully disclose what happened. The violation probably took grooming to get the person to trust you. This grooming is part of the violation. In detail, outline the step-by-step process involved in your victimization. When you get to the actual act of violation, be careful not to write "and then I had sex with her." It may be more appropriate to use anatomical terms.

The truth of what you are going to be writing will be the most rigorously honest and most painful work in the entire process of your recovery. This exercise is essential to help you own and accept these victimizations and may help rid you of any criminal thinking. The victims were in no sense to blame and deep down you know this, so be as responsible for your behavior as possible. Do this exercise for each victim. If you don't know their name or age, guess their age and give them a name.

EXERCISE # 92

EMPATHY LETTER

You have completed some of the hardest work yet and if you have committed violations against others, you are well aware of the guilt and shame you carry due to this choice of behavior. You need to go one step further in the healing process due to these violations.

Write the victim's name at the top of a piece of paper. After you have done this, begin to write to them as to how it must have felt to them spiritually, emotionally, physically and sexually to be victimized by you. Include how the event(s) probably hurt them for a very long time. After completing this part of the letter, you can write anything else you want to say to them in the rest of the letter. You can then read it out loud to them by imagining them in an empty chair next to you. You may experience a wide range of emotions at this point. If you feel safer having a support person or a therapist involved in this process please do so.

When you have finished one of your letters, wait a day or two and then go on to the next letter. This process may take a while, don't rush it. You and your recovery are worth every amount of effort you are expending during this phase of your freedom.

EXERCISE # 93

<u>SELF-FORGIVENESS</u>

After all the victim empathy letters are completed, there is still more to do. Again you are to be affirmed for the courage and commitment to your recovery that you have mustered up in order to face these very deep and sensitive issues in your life.

During the time of your acting out and possibly victimizing others, you may have a list of things that you would love to be forgiven of. The guilt, shame and fear can be overwhelming when you keep such a list inside of yourself.

Often you are the hardest of all on yourself. You may be limited in your ability to love and accept yourself as an addict. Hopefully by this time in your recovery there is a ray of love and hope for yourself.

In this exercise you have a letter to write also. This time the letter is to you. You are to write a letter to ask yourself to forgive yourself. You know what you did and what you need to be forgiven for specifically. This process can help you begin a dialog of self-forgiveness for what you have done in your past. This can open the door later to truly being free from past pain and guilt.

This letter can be as long as you like. Take your time as you work through this letter. Your recovery is worth it. You can write this letter below on the lines provided or on a separate piece of paper.

_____

_____

_____

_____

_____

_____

_____

_____

EXERCISE # 94

<u>BUT GOD...</u>

There is one final exercise to complete in order to finish the victimizing healing process and that is your relationship to God. This exercise is similar to the one you just completed. Imagine God in a chair in front of you and ask God to forgive you of the things you have done. After you have asked for forgiveness of God, imagine switching chairs with Him. You are now to respond as God would. Decide how you want Him to respond to this request of forgiveness you just heard.

After God (that is you) said what He needed to, switch back to the first chair. In this chair, respond to what God said to you.

In the space below, write out God's response and your response back to God.

_____

_____

_____

_____

_____

_____

_____

_____

_____

_____

EXERCISE # 95

STEP EIGHT

*"Made a list of all persons we have harmed
and became willing to make amends to them all."*

Step Eight is yet another one that involves journaling. This step is quite straightforward. List on a piece of paper those you feel you have harmed especially as it pertains to your sexual addiction.

In the midst of your addiction, you were medicated, unaware of what you were doing and whom you were hurting. Now in your recovery, you are sober enough to know that your acting out has a price to pay. If you need help with this list, consult your Fourth Step. Most people on your "bad" list column will qualify for this list in Step Eight.

After you make your list, put a percentage next to it representing how currently ready you are to make an amend to this person, (i.e. Joe - 75%). Review your list regularly until all people on your list have 100% next to them. This exercise may take prayer and reflection until all people have a 100% next to their name. This Step is just to move us to be "willing".

Behaviors that support Step Eight are as follows.

BEHAVIORS	YES	NO
1. A list of persons harmed	_____	_____
2. Percentages that increase	_____	_____
3. Prayer and reflection	_____	_____
4. Discussion with support people over difficult issues	_____	_____

126

EXERCISE # 96

STEP NINE

***"Made direct amends to such people wherever possible,
except when to do so would injure them or others."***

This step does take into consideration those to whom your direct amends "may" injure. This part of the step is not a loophole so that you don't have to make an amend. If you feel you have such a situation, talk to two people who have completed their Step Eight and/or a therapist and if they agree with you, then this is probably a legitimate situation not to give an amend.

The rest of this step is quite simple to do. With the list you have from Step Nine, write next to each name the most direct approach to do your amend whether face to face, by phone call or letter (i.e., Joe, person several states away - phone call). The issue of contacting past sexual partners should be discussed with your sponsor or a therapist before contacting them.

When your list of people with contact methods are complete, you are ready to start. Writing down the date you completed your amend is helpful to keep you motivated to finish the entire list. A complete entry might look like this.

Joe: Father-in-law   Face to face method   Date completed: 01-12-00

Behaviors that support a Step Nine are as follows.

BEHAVIORS	**YES**	**NO**
1. List of people	_____	_____
2. Method of contact list	_____	_____
3. Discussion with sponsor/therapist about those you have questions about contacting	_____	_____
4. Regular progress	_____	_____
5. A completed list	_____	_____

PART THREE:

MAINTAINING FREEDOM TECHNIQUES

EXERCISE # 97

STEP TEN

"Continued to take personal inventory and when we were wrong, promptly admit it."

Continuing to do anything means that you have already started doing something. Congratulations! You are entering what some call the "maintenance" part of the Twelve Step process. Step Ten does not allow you to have secrets in your closet especially now that you put all your time and energy into cleaning it out.

Keeping a healthy recovery is a discipline. In this step, journalling a daily personal inventory is your tool to make sure that you are "staying clean" with yourself and others. In this step, you will reflect daily with yourself and ask, "is there anything I did today that I know wasn't honest or right." If so, make an amend to this person.

Those who are married or have children will find a lot of opportunities to practice your recovery and stay humble. When this process is integrated, it can provide a lifestyle of honesty for your own well being and integrity with others.

Behaviors that support a Step Ten are as follows.

BEHAVIORS	YES	NO
1. Daily reflection	____	____
2. Check off your findings for the day	____	____
3. Check off daily any offenses made (remember, "promptly")	____	____
4. Ongoing discussions about steps with sponsor or therapist	____	____

EXERCISE # 98

DEVELOPING NEW INTERESTS

Exercise

The tool of "physical exercise" can help several ways in recovery. Exercise releases natural opiates to the brain. This gives your brain an alternative way (other than acting-out sexually) to get it's "brain cookies." Regular exercise can reactivate a neurological pathway you had as a teenager and can help shift the brain's dependency of acting out sexually as it's primary "brain cookie" and rely more on exercise.

Secondly, exercise can help you release stress. This release may help you stay more focused in your recovery. Exercise can help you maintain a more positive outlook and have increased energy to work on recovery issues such as relating to others.

Thirdly, exercise when consistent, can give you a sense of accomplishment. This can help your self-esteem. The more you like yourself, the less likely you are to want to hurt yourself, including acting-out sexually.

Exercise is an essential part of recovery. In treatment centers for addiction, trained professionals get clients to exercise regularly while in treatment. As in all exercise, it starts off slow. Get your doctor's approval and above all, make it fun. I personally find 20 to 30 minutes of aerobic activity makes a significant difference.

Make a list of your exercise activities including the days of the week and the times you will exercise for the next 90 days. If you need someone to be accountable to, write down that person's name.

NOTE: Exercise can be combined with re-socializing yourself also. There are clubs for running, biking, volleyball, and softball leagues, etc. Check your yellow pages or call and visit your local YMCA.

Developing New Interests

As a sex addict, you may have slowly drifted into a small isolated world. In this isolated world was your primary fix (wife), children, work acquaintances and your addiction, and rarely in that order. I can't tell you how many addicts have told me that their thoughts and behaviors are primarily motivated by their addiction. This does not leave much time and money for the pursuit of things you used to do. As your addiction takes over your life, usually hobbies and relationships, go to the side, unless they were a cover up for your sexual addiction or a way to get access to your victims.

(Cont'd next page)

In recovery as you move past the survival stage, you will need to have a balance of social and personal activities. There is no magical way to make this happen. First, make a list of activities you used to enjoy and a list of things you think you might enjoy. Secondly, find out where you have to go to do these activities. Thirdly, go a few times and if you like it, add this activity as part of your life recovery plan.

EXERCISE # 99

STEP ELEVEN

"Sought through prayer and meditation to improve our conscious contact with God as we understood Him, praying only for the knowledge of His will for us and the power to carry that out."

Prayer has been said to be "talking to God" whether it be requests, petitions, complaints, feelings and whatever other thoughts you might want to share in your personal relationship with God. Meditation is the point after you have quieted down and actually listen to hear what is on His mind. Both prayer and meditation are important. You have already established some type of relationship with God. This is a time to strengthen or improve that relationship.

Asking God for His will may be unfamiliar at first but as you do it, you will realize His will always has your best interest at heart. He is a Father who loves you dearly. Since He takes the time and energy to communicate His will for you, it is my experience that He will give you the Power to carry it out. This may be unfamiliar at first, but this step allows you to practice hearing and following through with God. This can open up a whole new aspect to your spiritual life that will enhance your freedom from sexual addiction.

Behaviors that support a Step Eleven are as follows.

BEHAVIORS   **YES   NO**

1. A regular time with God   _____ _____

2. Journal what God is saying   _____ _____

3. Keeping track of following God's will and the results   _____ _____

4. Increased reading and discussing spiritual matters   _____ _____

EXERCISE # 100

<u>STEP TWELVE</u>

"Having had a spiritual awakening as a result of these steps,
we tried to carry this message to others
and to practice these principles in all our affairs."

I enjoy getting results, no matter what the activity or area of my life that I am working on, especially when the results are obvious. Your recovery has included a lot of hard emotional work and self-discovery. It is through these steps that you had a "spiritual awakening."

You now have something to share. I was a sex addict, damaging myself and others and now, through this process, I am not acting-out and for the first time am able to look at others and myself. There are people throughout your life who will need this message of hope. When these people come across your path, through whatever circumstances, share your strength, hope and experience with them.

To be able to practice honesty, integrity, and spirituality is a gift that your recovery from sex addiction has given to you. To keep sobriety is to keep practicing what you learned in your steps that have given you abstinence from your behavior.

Behaviors that support Step Twelve are as follows.

BEHAVIOR	<u>Yes</u>	<u>No</u>
1. Continued abstinence from acting-out	_____	_____
2. Continued honesty and integrity	_____	_____
3. Continued amends when they are due	_____	_____
4. A life-style of healthy relationships	_____	_____

EXERCISE # 101

GIVING IT AWAY

In a study of alcoholics who were followed for ten years by a researcher, he found that there were only two variables that set apart the recovering alcoholic still sober for ten years and the alcoholics who went back to drinking. One of the two variables that separated the successful recovering alcoholic from the unsuccessful was the successful recovering alcoholic regularly attended their 12 Step Support Group, Alcoholic Anonymous. The second variable was the fact that these successful recovering alcoholics sponsored people in AA. In a sense they were "giving it away." You will hear in support groups time and time again that, "to keep it, you have to give it away." This is now a scientific fact.

As you recover from sexual addiction, you will find great changes occurring in your life. Your return to sanity will probably affect all areas of your life spiritually, socially, and sexually.

If you would like to start a Freedom Group in your church, you can "give it away" to other members (sex addicts are in every church, guaranteed) and to those in your community. Many need freedom so badly that they will even go to a church group if it would help! You will see the Lord naturally send people to you who need your help. When their lives become as changed as yours, you will experience the same joy I see daily in my life. May God bless your journey toward freedom.

Dr. Doug

APPENDIX

APPENDIX A
FEELINGS EXERCISE

1. I feel (put feeling word here) when (put a present situation when you feel this).

2. I first remember feeling (put the same feeling word here) when (earliest occurrence of this feeling).

Abandoned	Battered	Considerate	Distrusted	Goofy
Abused	Beaten	Consumed	Disturbed	Grateful
Aching	Beautiful	Content	Dominated	Greedy
Accepted	Belligerent	Cool	Domineering	Grief
Accused	Belittled	Courageous	Doomed	Grim
Accepting	Bereaved	Courteous	Doubtful	Grimy
Admired	Betrayed	Coy	Dreadful	Grouchy
Adored	Bewildered	Crabby	Eager	Grumpy
Adventurous	Blamed	Cranky	Ecstatic	Hard
Affectionate	Blaming	Crazy	Edgy	Harried
Agony	Bonded	Creative	Edified	Hassled
Alienated	Bored	Critical	Elated	Healthy
Aloof	Bothered	Criticized	Embarrassed	Helpful
Aggravated	Brave	Cross	Empowered	Helpless
Agreeable	Breathless	Crushed	Empty	Hesitant
Aggressive	Bristling	Cuddly	Enraged	High
Alive	Broken-up	Curious	Enraptured	Hollow
Alone	Bruised	Cut	Enthusiastic	Honest
Alluring	Bubbly	Damned	Enticed	Hopeful
Amazed	Burdened	Dangerous	Esteemed	Hopeless
Amused	Burned	Daring	Exasperated	Horrified
Angry	Callous	Dead	Excited	Hostile
Anguished	Calm	Deceived	Exhilarated	Humiliated
Annoyed	Capable	Deceptive	Exposed	Hurried
Anxious	Captivated	Defensive	Fake	Hurt
Apart	Carefree	Delicate	Fascinated	Hyper
Apathetic	Careful	Delighted	Feisty	Ignorant
Apologetic	Careless	Demeaned	Ferocious	Ignored
Appreciated	Caring	Demoralized	Foolish	Immature
Appreciative	Cautious	Dependent	Forced	Impatient
Apprehensive	Certain	Depressed	Forceful	Important
Appropriate	Chased	Deprived	Forgiven	Impotent
Approved	Cheated	Deserted	Forgotten	Impressed
Argumentative	Cheerful	Desirable	Free	Incompetent
Aroused	Childlike	Desired	Friendly	Incomplete
Astonished	Choked-up	Despair	Frightened	Independent
Assertive	Close	Despondent	Frustrated	Insecure
Attached	Cold	Destroyed	Full	Innocent
Attacked	Comfortable	Different	Funny	Insignificant
Attentive	Comforted	Dirty	Furious	Insincere
Attractive	Competent	Disenchanted	Gay	Isolated
Aware	Competitive	Disgusted	Generous	Inspired
Awestruck	Complacent	Disinterested	Gentle	Insulted
Badgered	Complete	Dispirited	Genuine	Interested
Baited	Confident	Distressed	Giddy	Intimate
Bashful	Confused	Distrustful	Giving	Intolerant

Involved	Pleased	Separated	Tormented
Irate	Positive	Sensuous	Torn
Irrational	Powerless	Sexy	Tortured
Irked	Present	Shattered	Touched
Irresponsible	Precious	Shocked	Trapped
Irritable	Pressured	Shot down	Tremendous
Irritated	Pretty	Shy	Tricked
Isolated	Proud	Sickened	Trusted
Jealous	Pulled apart	Silly	Trustful
Jittery	Put down	Sincere	Trusting
Joyous	Puzzled	Sinking	Ugly
Lively	Quarrelsome	Smart	Unacceptable
Lonely	Queer	Smothered	Unapproachable
Loose	Quiet	Smug	Unaware
Lost	Raped	Sneaky	Uncertain
Loving	Ravished	Snowed	Uncomfortable
Low	Ravishing	Soft	Under control
Lucky	Real	Solid	Understanding
Lustful	Refreshed	Solitary	Understood
Mad	Regretful	Sorry	Undesirable
Maudlin	Rejected	Spacey	Unfriendly
Malicious	Rejuvenated	Special	Ungrateful
Mean	Rejecting	Spiteful	Unified
Miserable	Relaxed	Spontaneous	Unhappy
Misunderstood	Relieved	Squelched	Unimpressed
Moody	Remarkable	Starved	Unsafe
Morose	Remembered	Stiff	Unstable
Mournful	Removed	Stimulated	Upset
Mystified	Repulsed	Stifled	Uptight
Nasty	Repulsive	Strangled	Used
Nervous	Resentful	Strong	Useful
Nice	Resistant	Stubborn	Useless
Numb	Responsible	Stuck	Unworthy
Nurtured	Responsive	Stunned	Validated
Nuts	Repressed	Stupid	Valuable
Obsessed	Respected	Subdued	Valued
Offended	Restless	Submissive	Victorious
Open	Revolved	Successful	Violated
Ornery	Riled	Suffocated	Violent
Out of control	Rotten	Sure	Voluptuous
Overcome	Ruined	Sweet	Vulnerable
Overjoyed	Sad	Sympathy	Warm
Overpowered	Safe	Tainted	Wary
Overwhelmed	Satiated	Tearful	Weak
Pampered	Satisfied	Tender	Whipped
Panicked	Scared	Tense	Whole
Paralyzed	Scolded	Terrific	Wicked
Paranoid	Scorned	Terrified	Wild
Patient	Scrutinized	Thrilled	Willing
Peaceful	Secure	Ticked	Wiped out
Pensive	Seduced	Tickled	Wishful
Perceptive	Seductive	Tight	Withdrawn
Perturbed	Self-centered	Timid	Wonderful
Phony	Self-conscious	Tired	Worried
Pleasant	Selfish	Tolerant	Worthy

TIME/COST CARD

AGE	Hours In Addiction Weekly	Multiply by 260 (52wks x 5 yrs)	Hourly Rate At The Time	Total Dollar Amt.
15-20				
20-25				
25-30				
30-35				
35-40				
40-45				
45-50				
50-55				
55-60				
60+				

Total time in money value_____

OTHER COSTS

Prostitutes _____

Phone Sex _____

Internet _____

Therapy _____

Guilt Offerings _____

Pornography _____

Legal Fees _____

Divorce/Child Support _____

Lost business/educ.opport. _____

Other _____

Subtotal_____   **OVER ALL TOTAL COST** _____

The Twelve Steps of Alcoholics Anonymous

1. We admitted we were powerless over alcohol--that our lives had become unmanageable.

2. Came to believe that a Power greater than ourselves could restore us to sanity.

3. Made a decision to turn our will and our lives over to the care of God as we understood Him.

4. Made a searching and fearless moral inventory of ourselves.

5. Admitted to God, to ourselves, and to another human being the exact nature of our wrongs.

6. Were entirely ready to have God remove all these defects of character.

7. Humbly asked Him to remove our shortcomings.

8. Made a list of all people we had harmed, and became willing to make amends to them all.

9. Made direct amends to such people wherever possible, except when to do so would injure them or others.

10. Continued to take personal inventory, and when we were wrong, promptly admitted it.

11. Sought through prayer and meditation to improve our conscious contact with God as we understood Him, praying only for knowledge of His will for us and the power to carry that out.

12. Having had a spiritual awakening as the result of these steps, we tried to carry this message to others and to practice these principles in all our affairs.

The Twelve Steps of Alcoholics Anonymous
Adapted for Sexual Addicts

1. We admitted we were powerless over our sexual addiction--that our lives had become unmanageable.

2. Came to believe that a Power greater than ourselves could restore us to sanity.

3. Made a decision to turn our will and our lives over to the care of God as we understood Him.

4. Made a searching and fearless moral inventory of ourselves.

5. Admitted to God, to ourselves, and to another human being the exact nature of our wrongs.

6. Were entirely ready to have God remove all these defects of character.

7. Humbly asked Him to remove our shortcomings.

8. Made a list of all people we had harmed, and became willing to make amends to them all.

9. Made direct amends to such people wherever possible, except when to do so would injure them or others.

10. Continued to take personal inventory, and when we were wrong, promptly admitted it.

11. Sought through prayer and meditation to improve our conscious contact with God as we understood Him, praying only for knowledge of His will for us and the power to carry that out.

12. Having had a spiritual awakening as the result of these steps, we tried to carry this message to others and to practice these principles in all our affairs.

SUPPORT GROUPS

SEX ADDICTION

Sex Addicts Anonymous
P.O. Box 70949
Houston, TX 77270
(713) 869-4902

Sexaholics Anonymous
P.O. Box 111910
Nashville, TN 37222-1910
(615) 331-6901

Sexual Compulsives
Anonymous (SCA)
Old Chelsea Station,
P.O. Box 1585
New York, NY 10013-0935
1-800-977-HEAL

Sex and Love Addicts Anonymous (SLAA)
P.O. Box 338, Norwood,
Boston, MA 02062
(617) 781-255-8825

Sexual Recovery Anonymous
(SRA),
PO Box 73,Planetarium
Station,
New York, NY 10024
(212) 340-4650 or:
PO Box 72044
Burnaby, BC V5H4PQ Canada
(604) 290-9382

FOR THE WIFE OR FAMILY MEMBER

Co-dependents of Sex
Addicts (COSA),
P.O. Box 14537
Minneapolis, MN 55414,
(612) 537-6904

S-Anon International
Family Groups
P.O. Box 111242
Nashville, TN 37222-1242
(615) 833-3152

Co-SLAA
P.O. Box 614
Brookline, MA 02146

Recovering Couples
Anonymous (RCA)
P.O. Box 11872
St. Louis, MO 63105
(314) 830-2600

SEXUAL TRAUMA SURVIVORS

Survivors of Incest Anonymous (SIA)
P.O. Box 21817
Baltimore, MD 21222
(410) 282-3400

Incest Survivors Anonymous
(ISA)
P.O. Box 17245
Long Beach, CA 90807

Sexual Assault Recovery
Anonymous (SARA Society),
P.O. Box 16
Surrey, British Columbia,
V35 424, Canada
(604) 584-2626

MATERIAL DESCRIPTIONS

Sex Addiction Materials

***The Final Freedom,* by Weiss--Audio $35.00/Book $22.95** In addition to informing sex addicts about sex addiction, this product gives hope for recovery. This book underscores the biological and psychological aspects of sex addiction and gives a road map to recovery. Many have attested to successful recovery from this product alone.

***Steps to Freedom: A Christian 12 Step Guide,* by Weiss--$14.95** This workbook is a thorough interaction with the Twelve Steps of recovery from a Christian perspective. Can be used in Twelve Step study groups, or individually.

VIDEO THERAPY, by Weiss--Session #1 @ $69.95, Sessions #2-6 @ $39.95 each
  Session #1 How Did I Get This Way?, by Weiss--90 min. This is the same intake session you would have with Dr. Weiss in his office. You will identify how you became a sex addict (biologically, psychological, or trauma based) and if you are both a sex addict and anorexic and how this all impacts your treatment.
  Session #2 How To Get and Stay Clean This is a very impacting video. Dr. Weiss shares techniques that work toward recovery that are tried and tested. Discussed is how to win and how to lose your recovery.
  Session #3 Sexual Abuse Over 80% of sex addicts report being sexually abused. This is a very practical and educational video. Dealing with sexual abuse issues in treatment expedites your personal recovery from sex addiction.
  Session #4 Dealing with Family of Origin Many of us have family of origin issues. Dealing with Mom and Dad's neglect or abuse whether intentional or not is important during your recovery. This tape walks you through exercises Dr. Weiss uses in his office to facilitate healing from family of origin issues.
  Session #5 Guilt and Shame Sex addicts carry guilt of events participated in as well as shame of who the he has become. Your destiny without guilt and shame can be trans forming. Dr. Weiss has you practically deal with these important issues in this video.
  Session #6 The Christian Sex Addict--$39.95 Christians suffer from sexual addiction as well as other people. This tape is full of biblical examples of sex addiction and has biblical principles for recovery. If you are a Christian sex addict, this will not only facilitate your recovery, it will build your faith. God still has a plan for you! This video can help you get and stay free from your sexual addiction.

***Sexual Anorexia,* by Weiss--90 min. Video $69.95** Sexual anorexia paralyzes sex addicts from having intimate relationships with others. This video will provide practical steps to stop withholding behaviors and begin intimacy in present and future relationships.
***She Has A Secret: Understanding Female Sexual Addiction,* by Weiss--$14.95** This leading book on female sexual addiction combines true stories of female addicts with the most recent research to understand female sex addicts. This book is a must for any woman struggling with sexual addiction.

Partner's Materials

***Partner's Recovery Guide: 100 Empowering Exercises,* by Weiss--$39.95**
This is the most practical workbook for partners and was conceived through many years of successfully treating partners of sex addicts.

***Now That I Know, What Should I Do?,* by Weiss--$69.95** This 90 minute video answers the ten most frequently asked questions by partners just finding out about their spouse's sexual addiction. The need for counseling is significantly reduced by listening to this video.

***Women Who Love Sex Addicts,* by Weiss--$14.95** This book discusses what the wife can do to help cope in her relationship with a sex addict. Wives of sex addicts will find this book both informative and comforting.

***Beyond Love:12 Step Recovery Guide for Partners,* by Weiss--$14.95** This is a wife's interactive workbook to gain insight and strength through the Twelve Steps. This book can be used alone or as a group step-study workbook.

***How to Love When it Hurts So Bad,* by Weiss-- $38.00** This 4-tape audio series and workbook deals with the wife's issues in living with an addict. This has a religious focus and gives biblical answers to boundaries, tough love, and how to love an addict the way God does. It has a twelve-step approach.

Other Materials

Good Enough to Wait--by Weiss--$39.95 This 60 minute video is the Christian sex talk for teenagers for the 21st Century. Dr. Weiss combines the best scriptural teaching with years of research in the field of sexuality. This video comes with a commitment card (which researchers have found to profoundly increase the chances of waiting till marriage) and work booklet. Youth Pastors in addition to parents will also greatly benefit from this video presentation.

Good Enough To Wait--$12.95/T-Shirt Description: On front: GOOD ENOUGH, On Back: TO WAIT (picture of a young couple in the background/soft gray) All words in purple. Available in sizes L, XL

***Pathways To Intimacy,* by Weiss Robison, Evans--$35.00/5 Audios** This audio series presents solutions to gaining intimacy in the marriage relationship. Nuggets of information are gleaned from national television host James Robison, author Douglas Weiss, Ph.D. and Debra Evans. This is a great road map for couples wanting more intimacy out of their relationship.

ORDER FORM

ITEM	QUANTITY	PRICE	TOTAL

VIDEOS/AUDIOS

ITEM	QUANTITY	PRICE	TOTAL
Video Therapy: *Session #1 How Did I Get This Way?*	_____	$69.95	_____
Session #2 How To Get and Stay Clean	_____	39.95	_____
NEW! *Session #3 Sexual Abuse*	_____	39.95	_____
Session #4 Dealing with Family of Origin	_____	39.95	_____
Session #5 Guilt and Shame	_____	39.95	_____
Session #6 The Christian Sex Addict	_____	39.95	_____
Sexual Anorexia, (90 min Video) by Weiss	_____	69.95	_____
The Final Freedom, (5 audios), Weiss	_____	35.00	_____
Good Enough To Wait, (1hr. Video) by Weiss	_____	39.95	_____
Good Enough To Wait, (T-Shirt) XL, L sizes	_____	12.95	_____
Now That I Know, What Should I Do?, Weiss (90 min Video)	_____	69.95	_____
How To Love When It Hurts So Bad, (4 audios/1 wkbk) Weiss	_____	38.00	_____
Pathways To Intimacy, (Audio Series)	_____	35.00	_____

BOOKS/WORKBOOKS

ITEM	QUANTITY	PRICE	TOTAL
The Final Freedom, (Book) by Weiss	_____	22.95	_____
101 Freedom Exercises for Sex Addiction Recovery, by Weiss	_____	39.95	_____
Steps to Freedom, by Weiss	_____	14.95	_____
Faithful and True, by Laaser	_____	14.95	_____
Hope and Recovery, by Hazelden	_____	14.95	_____
Sex and Love, by Griffin-Shelley	_____	29.95	_____
Sex, Lies and Forgiveness, by Schneider	_____	14.95	_____
Partner's Recovery Guide: 100 Empowering Exercises, Weiss	_____	39.95	_____
Beyond Love, by Weiss	_____	14.95	_____
Women Who Love Sex Addicts, by Weiss & DeBusk	_____	14.95	_____
Affair of the Mind, by Hall	_____	14.95	_____
She Has a Secret: Understanding female sex addiction, Weiss	_____	14.95	_____

Sub Total _____

8.25% Sales Tax (in Texas only) _____

Shipping/Handling-add $3 + .50 for each additional item (in USA) _____

Shipping/Handling-add $6 + $1 for each additional item (outside USA) _____

Total _____

To order: 817-377-4278

VISA/MC/DISCOVER # _____ EXP DATE _____

NAME _____ SIGNATURE _____

ADDRESS _____ CITY _____

STATE _____ ZIP CODE _____ PHONE (___)_____

MAIL: Heart to Heart Counseling Centers, P.O. Box 16716, Fort Worth, TX, 76162-0716

E-MAIL: heart2heart@xc.org   Website: www.sexaddict.com

(Make Checks payable to Heart to Heart Counseling Center)

FREEDOM GROUPS

What are Freedom Groups?

Freedom Groups are Christ-based support groups for people wanting freedom from being sexually driven.

How do they work?

One man impressed by the Holy Spirit who wants to assist in helping others get freedom from being sexually driven asks his pastor to sponsor this ministry. This *pointman* will be the contact person for the church. The church will refer people who feel sexually driven to the *pointman*. This *pointman* will meet with those desiring help and will cover the *Freedom Principles* and *Freedom Covenant* with them. Once the person agrees to the *Freedom Principles* and *Freedom Covenant*, he is given the group location and time.

Freedom Group Roles

1. The *pointman* serves as contact person for anyone to be brought into the group. This is to protect the group from someone just dropping in on the group. The point man can serve for an indefinite amount of time but should be reconsidered after one year of service.
2. The *chairperson* of the meeting is responsible to start the meeting by asking the pointman if any new people need to make a Freedom Covenant. If there are no new Freedom Covenants to be addressed, the chairperson starts the introductions and chooses the topic for the group discussion. The chairperson serves the group for a maximum of 8 weeks. At that time someone else volunteers to chair the meeting.

Freedom Principles-For the First 100 Days of Recovery

1. Pray: Pray in the morning asking Jesus to keep you free today.
2. Read: Read the Bible and read freedom-related material.
3. Call: Call someone in your group and check in with that person at the beginning of each day.
4. Meetings: Attend every meeting possible.
5. Pray: Pray in the evening thanking God for keeping you free today.

One-Year Freedom Covenant

1. The members of the Freedom Group covenant to total confidentiality of all group members and discussions held during group meetings.
2. Members covenant to attend the Freedom Group for one year and to work through the Freedom Materials and report progress to the group.
3. Members covenant to keep the Freedom Principles for the first 100 days of their jour ney toward freedom.

Freedom Meetings

1. Any new members are introduced by the pointman and are asked to verbalize the Freedom Covenant to the group in the first person. (Example: I covenant to...)
2. Introductions: Beginning with the chairperson of the meeting, introductions are done as follows: The chairperson introduces himself, shares his feelings, shares his boundaries and length of time free from those behaviors.

(Example: "My name is John. I feel frustrated and alone. My boundaries to stay free are no pornography, bookstores, and no sex outside of marriage. I worked on Exercises #5-#7 in my 101 Freedom Exercises workbook and made four pages of progress on my Steps to Freedom workbook since our last meeting. I have been free for 3 weeks.")

3. The *chairperson* chooses a topic related to staying free from being sexually driven that the group discusses. Each member can share without feedback from the group, unless feedback is specifically asked for by the sharing member.
4. Honest Time: Group members pair off into 2-3 members and discuss thoughts, behaviors, struggles, and successes since the last meeting (James 5:16).
5. Closing Prayer: Group members get back together and repeat the Lord's Prayer together.

Freedom Group Materials

1. *The Final Freedom: Pioneering Sex Addiction Recovery*
2. *101 Freedom Exercises: A Christian Guide To Sex Addiction Recovery -*
3. *Steps To Freedom: A Christian 12-Step Guide For Sexual Addiction*

Freedom Group Topics for Discussion

Triggers	Honesty
Fear	Hope
Bottom Lines	Relapse
Control	H.A.L.T.
Steps 1-12	Boundaries
Prayer	Maximized Thinking
Recovery Rituals	Feelings
Anger	Dangerous Dabbling
Fun	Father Issues
Sexual Abuse	Grooming Victims
Objectifying	Accountability
Discipline	Acts of Love
My Calling	My Future
Daily Struggles	Dangerous Places
What Works	Dating My Wife
Control	Male Friends
Humility	Turning It Over
One Day at a Time	My Daily God Time
My Worst Moment	The Gift of Recovery
Breaking the Curse for My Children	Exercise
Addictions in My Family	God's Grace
What God Is Doing	Intimacy

...And any other topic the chairperson feels is appropriate. Remember, don't be graphic, be honest!

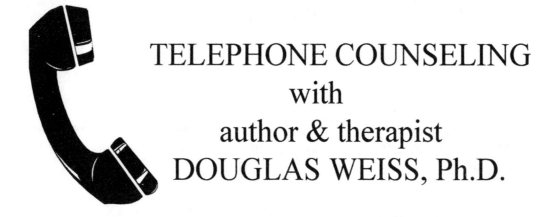

TELEPHONE COUNSELING
with
author & therapist
DOUGLAS WEISS, Ph.D.

Dear Reader,

We are happy to introduce you to the opportunity of telephone counseling with Douglas Weiss at Heart to Heart Counseling Centers. Counseling is provided for those having issues with sexual addiction, wives of sex addicts, victims of sexual trauma and marital issues. As you work through the *101 Freedom Exercises*, and you have some concerns or issues you would like professional help with, call Heart to Heart Counseling Centers. All telephone counseling is strictly confidential.

To schedule a telephone appointment with Dr. Douglas Weiss, **call 817-377-4278**. Telephone appointments are available Mon - Wed 8:00 a.m. to 7:00 p.m. central time. When you call to schedule your appointment, you will be given a **toll-free number** (within USA). Call the toll-free number at the time of your scheduled appointment. We will need 24 hours notice for changes in appointments or cancellations otherwise you will be billed for your appointment.

Counseling costs are $125.00 per hour. We accept Mastercard, VISA, American Express or Discover, or you may send a check in advance of your scheduled appointment. We look forward to hearing from you.

3-DAY INTENSIVE SCHEDULE
for 2000
with Douglas Weiss, Ph.D.
Fort Worth, Texas

Our 3-day Intensive workshops are a huge success. Couples receive 3 hours (individuals 2 1/2 hrs.) per day of personal counseling with Dr. Weiss. Support groups are also available during the evening. The following are Intensive dates available.

Individual Intensive Dates

Jan. 3-5	July 17-19
Jan. 17-19	July 31-Aug 2
Jan. 31-Feb.2	Aug 14-16
Feb 14-16	Sept.4-6
Feb 28-Mar 1	Sept. 18-20
Mar 13-15	Oct. 2-4
April 3-5	Oct. 16-18
April 17-19	Nov. 6-8
May 1-3	Nov. 20-22
May 15-17	Dec. 4-6
June 5-7	Dec. 13-20
June 19-21	Dec. 18-20

Couple Intensive Dates

Jan. 10-12	July 10-12
Jan. 24-26	July 24-26
Feb 7-9	Aug 7-Aug 9
Feb 21-23	Aug 21-23
Mar 6-8	Sept. 11-13
Mar 20-22	Sept.25-27
April 10-12	Oct. 9-11
April 24-26	Oct. 23-25
May 8-10	Nov. 13-15
May 22-24	Nov. 27-29
June 12-14	Dec. 11-13

Cost: $950/Individual Pre-paid*
         $1,200/Couple Pre-paid*

*Does not include travel, hotel or food
Call for hotel and activity packets

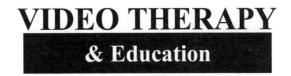

VIDEO THERAPY
& Education

By Douglas Weiss, Ph.D.

Dr. Weiss has put together his valuable sex addiction therapy & education into 6 **NEW** videos!

Video Session #1:   **How Did I Get This Way? (90 Min)**

Video Session #2:   **How To Get and Stay Clean. Preventing relapses!**

Video Session #3:   **Sexual Abuse: Living beyond the pain**

Video Session #4:   **Dealing with Family of Origin Issues**

Video Session #5:   **Guilt and Shame: Living without the voices**

Video Session #6:   **The Christian Sex Addict: The Biblical perspective**

WHY VIDEO THERAPY AND EDUCATION???

❑   **Is it hard to find a local therapist who understands sex addiction?**

❑   **Do you want help NOW without waiting for an appointment?**

❑   **Would you like the confidentiality of counseling in the privacy of your home?**

❑   **Are you uncomfortable talking to a therapist about your sexual addiction?**

❑   **Where can you get counseling by a national expert for these prices?**

The most affordable way to get this much information!

Join us

On The Internet

www.sexaddict.com

√   free newsletter for addicts

√   free newsletter for wives

√   research/books/videos and more

√   download video therapy sessions
      instantly!!